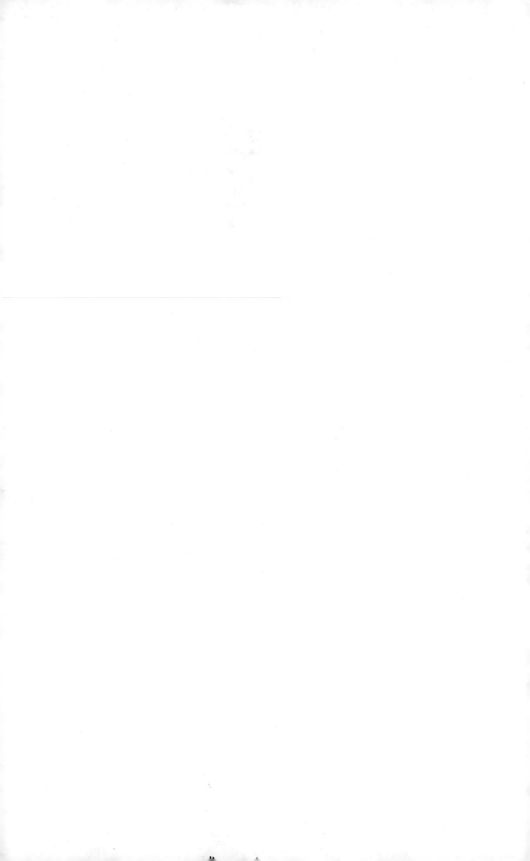

Integrating Evidence into Practice for Impact

Editors

DEBRA D. MARK
MARITA G. TITLER
RENE'E W. LATIMER

NURSING CLINICS
OF NORTH AMERICA

www.nursing.theclinics.com

Consulting Editor
STEPHEN D. KRAU

September 2014 • Volume 49 • Number 3

ELSEVIER

1600 John F. Kennedy Boulevard • Suite 1800 • Philadelphia, Pennsylvania, 19103-2899

http://www.theclinics.com

NURSING CLINICS OF NORTH AMERICA Volume 49, Number 3
September 2014 ISSN 0029-6465, ISBN-13: 978-0-323-32333-8

Editor: Kerry Holland
Developmental Editor: Casey Jackson

Nursing Clinics of North America (ISSN 0029-6465) is published quarterly by Elsevier Inc., 360 Park Avenue South, New York, NY 10010-1710. Months of issue are March, June, September, and December. Periodicals postage paid at New York, NY and additional mailing offices. Subscription price per year is, $150.00 (US individuals), $400.00 (US institutions), $275.00 (international individuals), $488.00 (international institutions), $220.00 (Canadian individuals), $488.00 (Canadian institutions), $85.00 (US students), and $135.00 (international students). To receive student/resident rate, orders must be accompanied by name of affiliated institution, date of term, and the signature of program/residency coordinator on institution letterhead. Orders will be billed at individual rate until proof of status is received. Foreign air speed delivery is included in all *Clinics* subscription prices. All prices are subject to change without notice. **POSTMASTER:** Send address changes to *Nursing Clinics*, Elsevier Health Sciences Division, Subscription Customer Service, 3251 Riverport Lane, Maryland Heights, MO 63043. **Customer Service: Telephone: 1-800-654-2452** (U.S. and Canada); **1-314-447-8871 (outside U.S. and Canada). Fax: 1-314-447-8029. E-mail: journalscustomerservice-usa@elsevier.com** (for print support) and **journalsonlinesupport-usa@elsevier.com** (for online support).

Nursing Clinics of North America is covered in *EMBASE/Excerpta Medica, MEDLINE/PubMed (Index Medicus), Social Sciences Citation Index, Current Contents, ASCA, Cumulative Index to Nursing, RNdex Top 100,* and Allied Health Literature and International Nursing Index (INI).

Printed in the United States of America.

Contributors

CONSULTING EDITOR

STEPHEN D. KRAU, PhD, RN, CNE
Associate Professor, Vanderbilt University Medical Center School of Nursing, Nashville, Tennessee

EDITORS

DEBRA D. MARK, PhD, RN
Nurse Researcher, Hawai'i State Center for Nursing; Assistant Professor, University of Hawai'i School of Nursing & Dental Hygiene, Honolulu, Hawaii

MARITA G. TITLER, PhD, RN, FAAN
Professor and Associate Dean for Practice and Clinical Scholarship; Rhetaugh Dumas Endowed Chair; Department Chair, Systems Leadership and Effectiveness Science, University of Michigan School of Nursing, Ann Arbor, Michigan

RENE'E W. LATIMER, MPH, MSN, RN
Queen Emma Nursing Institute, Director, The Queen's Medical Center, Honolulu, Hawaii

AUTHORS

MICHELLE AEBERSOLD, PhD, RN
Clinical Assistant Professor, Director of the Clinical Learning Center, Division of Systems Leadership and Effectiveness Science, University of Michigan School of Nursing, Ann Arbor, Michigan

FLORENCE AGOS, BSN, RN
Clinical Operations Manager, Orthopedic Surgery Unit and Surgical Short Stay Unit, The Queen's Medical Center, Honolulu, Hawaii

SUSAN BANKHEAD, MSN, DNP
Clinical Service Line Manager, Pediatric Intensive Care Unit, Kapiolani Medical Center for Women & Children, Honolulu, Hawaii; Director of Pediatrics and PICU, Eastern Idaho Regional Medical Center, Idaho Falls, Idaho

JULIET G. BENIGA, BSN, RN, CNRN, CCRN
Staff Nurse IV, Neuroscience Institute, Neuroscience Intensive Care Unit, The Queen's Medical Center, Honolulu, Hawaii

DEBORAH BRANSFORD, BSN, RN
Certified Diabetes Educator and Evidence-based Practice Mentor, Patient Care Consulting Services, The Queen's Medical Center, Honolulu, Hawaii

KATIE CARTER, RNC-NIC, BSN
Staff Nurse, Neonatal Intensive Care Unit, Tripler Army Medical Center, Honolulu, Hawaii

KOLEA CHONG, BSN, CCRN
Pediatric Intensive Care Unit, Kapiolani Medical Center for Women & Children, Honolulu, Hawaii

REBECCA COLE, RN, BS
Performance Improvement Coordinator, Emergency Department, The Queen's Medical Center, Honolulu, Hawaii

KATHLEEN DOI, APRN, MS, CNS
Clinical Nurse Specialist, Pain Service, Kaiser Moanalua Medical Center, Honolulu, Hawaii

MARYLINE DOLOR, BSN, RN
QET 8DH/Ortho Joint Trauma, The Queen's Medical Center, Honolulu, Hawaii

CAPTAIN ALLISON FERRO, RN-BC
Clinical Nurse Officer in Charge, Medical Oncology, Tripler Army Medical Center, Honolulu, Hawaii

MAIMONA GHOWS, MD
Intensivist, SICU, The Queen's Medical Center, Honolulu, Hawaii

GREGORY GIBBONS, BSN, CCRN, CPAN, CAPA
Staff Nurse, Post Anesthesia Care Unit, Kaiser Moanalua Medical Center, Honolulu, Hawaii

MICHELE HADANO, MS, RN
QET 8DH/Ortho Joint Trauma, The Queen's Medical Center, Honolulu, Hawaii

LOIS HAN, BSN, RN, CCRN
Charge Nurse, SICU, The Queen's Medical Center, Honolulu, Hawaii

SUSAN B. HASSMILLER, PhD, RN, FAAN
Senior Adviser for Nursing, and Director, *The Future of Nursing: Campaign for Action*, Robert Wood Johnson Foundation, Princeton, New Jersey

ROSE K.L. HATA, MS, RN, APRN, CCRN, CCNS
Clinical Nurse Specialist, SICU, The Queen's Medical Center, Honolulu, Hawaii

LEILANI JEAN B. HILL, BSN, RN
Staff Nurse, The Queen's Medical Center, Honolulu, Hawaii

SALLY ISHIKAWA, RN, NHA, MPH, C-DONA
Chief Nurse Executive (Former), Leahi Hospital, Honolulu, Hawaii

KARA IZUMI, PharmD, BCPS, BCNSP
Clinical Pharmacist, SICU, The Queen's Medical Center, Honolulu, Hawaii

KATHERINE G. JOHNSON, MS, RN, APRN, CCRN, CNRN, CNS-BC
Clinical Nurse Specialist, Neuroscience Institute, The Queen's Medical Center, Honolulu, Hawaii

SALLY KAMAI, RN, MBA-HCM
Director, Clinical Improvement, Hawaii Pacific Health, Honolulu, Hawaii

RENE'E W. LATIMER, MPH, MSN, RN
Director, Queen Emma Nursing Institute, The Queen's Medical Center, Honolulu, Hawaii

VICKIE LAUBACH, RNC-NIC, MSN
Clinical Nurse Educator, Neonatal Intensive Care Unit, Tripler Army Medical Center, Honolulu, Hawaii

DEBRA D. MARK, PhD, RN
Nurse Researcher, Hawai'i State Center for Nursing; Assistant Professor, University of Hawai'i School of Nursing & Dental Hygiene, Honolulu, Hawaii

ASA MIYAHIRA, BSN, RN, CCRN
Staff Nurse, SICU, The Queen's Medical Center, Honolulu, Hawaii

FIRST LIEUTENANT KATRINA MULLENS, RN-BC
Staff Nurse, Medical Oncology, Tripler Army Medical Center, Honolulu, Hawaii

CHRISTYANNE PASSION, MSN, RN, CCRN
Staff Nurse, SICU, The Queen's Medical Center, Honolulu, Hawaii

CAPTAIN SETH RANDALL, RN
Discharge Advocate, Medical Oncology, Tripler Army Medical Center, Honolulu, Hawaii

CHRISTINA SACOCO, RN, MS
Director, Quality Assurance, Leahi Hospital, Honolulu, Hawaii

ROSANNE SHIMODA, RN
Staff Nurse, Preoperative Evaluation and Education Center, Kaiser Moanalua Medical Center, Honolulu, Hawaii

CASEY SHODA, BSN, RN
Staff Nurse, Surgical Short Stay Unit, The Queen's Medical Center, Honolulu, Hawaii

JILL SLADE, BSN, RN, CCRN
Nurse Manager, SICU, The Queen's Medical Center, Honolulu, Hawaii

VALERIE L. SONG, BA
Editor, Hawai'i State Center for Nursing, Honolulu, Hawaii

MARITA G. TITLER, PhD, RN, FAAN
Professor and Associate Dean for Practice and Clinical Scholarship; Rhetaugh Dumas Endowed Chair; Department Chair, Systems Leadership and Effectiveness Science, University of Michigan School of Nursing, Ann Arbor, Michigan

JOAN P. WHITE, MBA, RN
Project Coordinator, Hawai'i State Center for Nursing, Honolulu, Hawaii

PATRICIA WILHELM, RNC-NIC, PhD
Nurse Manager, Neonatal Intensive Care Unit, Tripler Army Medical Center, Honolulu, Hawaii

MIHAE YU, MD, FACS
Program Director, Surgical Critical Care Fellowship; Professor of Surgery, Department of Surgery; Medical Director of SICU, The Queen's Medical Center; Vice-Chair of Education, University of Hawaii, Honolulu, Hawaii

Contents

> Evidence-based practice and translation science are not interchangeable terms; EBP is the application of evidence in practice (the doing of EBP), whereas translation science is the study of implementation interventions, factors, and contextual variables that affect knowledge uptake and use in practices and communities. The use of collaborative networks such as the National Nursing Practice Network maximizes sharing of resources and knowledge about EBPs, an infrastructure for conducting multi-site translation studies, and a venue for large scale-up of EBP projects across multiple healthcare settings.

> Hawaii's innovative statewide evidence-based practice program facilitates practice change across multiple health care systems. The innovation eliminated duplicative efforts and provided resources, was compatible with the values of health care organizations, and had experience with a pilot program. Interpersonal and mass media communication promoted and embedded the practice change. Users included nurse champions with multidisciplinary team members. The rate of adoption varied across projects and, although resources seemed to be a major determinant of successful institutionalization, there does not seem to be a predictable pattern of successful project implementation.

> A descriptive study of risk factors for surgical site infection (SSI) in patients receiving total knee arthroplasty discovered an infection rate higher than the benchmark. Although no risk factors were significant predictors of SSI in this population, an important finding was that, despite a patient population with comorbid diabetes, a lack of standardized practice related to the identification and management of hyperglycemia was identified. These findings identified and validated an important practice issue and led to the continued commitment to improve glucose management. In this

way, a study was a trigger for improved nursing practice using evidence-based practice.

Perioperative hyperglycemia management is an important factor in reducing the risk of surgical site infections (SSIs) in all patients regardless of existing history of diabetes. Reduction of SSIs is one of the quality indicators reported by the National Healthcare Safety Networks of the Centers for Disease Control and Prevention (CDC). In 2009 and 2010, the orthopedic surgical unit had an increased number of SSIs above the CDC benchmark. This article describes the impact of an evidence-based practice standard for perioperative hyperglycemia management in the reduction of SSIs in patients having total hip and knee replacement surgery.

This article describes an evidence-based approach to decreasing the length of stay of inpatient adults on the medicine oncology ward of a large urban military medical center. A strong and diverse team was formed, which worked together for the length of the project. A formalized approach involving weekly discharge-planning meetings with a discharge advocate as the planner, coupled with solid documentation, was adopted. There was a decrease in the average length of stay on the inpatient wards, resulting in cost savings for the facility. This approach using strong evidence can overcome institutional challenges, with a positive impact on patient care.

The objective of this project was to reduce the number of failed extubations in the pediatric intensive care unit. This article describes extubation failures in the pediatric intensive care unit and the development and implementation of an extubation readiness protocol using the Iowa Model for Evidence-based Practice as a guideline. The Iowa Model consists of processes for implementing evidence into practice, such as critiquing and synthesizing the literature, identifying stakeholders, and recognizing triggers. The extubation protocol was developed excluding children with previous lung injury and/or neuromuscular conditions, which contribute to an increased risk and complexity of planned extubations.

Attempting to mitigate operational and structural noise is important in improving the outcomes of high-risk preterm infants. It was anticipated that a culture change in nursing behaviors to include "Quiet Time" would result in reducing the noise levels towards the National Recommended Safe Sound Level. This culture change alone was inadequate to meet

NRL. Both operational and structural changes were also required in order to provide a safer neurophysiological environment for the rest and growth of the neonate.

Pain identification of cognitively impaired elderly is very challenging. This project aimed to identify best practices for pain assessment in nursing home residents with cognitive impairment and to establish a standardized pain assessment guide to optimize nursing practice and resident outcomes. The Iowa Model of Evidence-Based Practice to Promote Quality of Care guided the project's process. Phase I of the project analyzed data gained from chart reviews on current practices of pain assessment, and Phase II used the results of Phase I to develop, implement, and evaluate an evidence-based practice standard for nursing assessment of pain for cognitively impaired residents.

A traumatic spinal cord injury is a catastrophic event associated with physiologic disruptions to the motor, sensory, cardiovascular, and respiratory systems. Respiratory complications are a common cause of morbidity and mortality in patients with acute cervical spinal cord injury and treatments must be initiated immediately. The longer it takes for a patient to receive pulmonary treatments and mobility activities, the higher the morbidity and mortality and the longer the length of stay. Disrupted pulmonary mechanics and respiratory complications are frequent and are influenced by the level of injury.

Evidence supports reducing the use of restraints and seclusion because these episodes can result in psychological harm or physical injury to patients and staff. The goal was to discover better, more therapeutic methods for managing agitated emergency department behavioral health patients to minimize the use of restraints and seclusion. Training in verbal de-escalation techniques and simulation practice were key strategies in providing staff with the necessary tools and knowledge to change their practice to one of trauma-informed care.

Ensuring adequate sleep for hospitalized patients is important for reducing stress, improving healing, and decreasing episodes of delirium. The purpose of this project was to implement a Sleep Program for stable patients in the surgical intensive care unit, thereby changing sleep management practices and ensuring quality of care using an evidence-based practice approach. Improving patient satisfaction with sleep by 28 percentage points may be attributed to a standardized process of providing a healing environment for patients to sleep.

Fever is a significant contributor to secondary brain insult and management is a challenge for the neurocritical care team. The absence of standardized guidelines likely contributes to poor surveillance and undertreatment of increased temperature. A need for practice change was identified and this evidence-based practice project was initiated to compile sufficient evidence to develop, implement, and evaluate a treatment guideline to manage fever and maintain normothermia in the neurocritical care population. Ongoing education, inclusion in staff annual competency, and staff update on compliance performance is essential to maintain and sustain the practice change achieved through this project.

As increasing numbers of the baby boomer generation seek health care, nursing staff educated in the evidence-based practice process can make significant contributions to successful patient outcomes. Health care providers who anticipate the approaching perfect storm in health care and thoughtfully plan, collaborate, and incorporate evidence-based practice methods will be well-prepared to improve the quality of care, realize cost savings, and meet the challenges ahead.

Simulation has become a necessary and integral part of education for prelicensure and ongoing education of health care practitioners. To guide this process, the Simulation Model for Improving Learner and Health Outcomes (SMILHO) model provides a framework to design the experience from a science of learning approach and links it to learner and health outcomes to add to the knowledge base. Much work has been done in this area, and the SMILHO model will support the future work needed to continue to create effective simulation-based learning experiences and move research from knowledge and skill evaluation to learner and health outcomes.

NURSING CLINICS OF NORTH AMERICA

Foreword

Evidence-based Practice: Another Passing Phrase, or Here to Stay?

 CrossMark

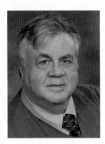

Stephen D. Krau, PhD, RN, CNE
Consulting Editor

A bell is no bell till you ring it. A song is no song till you sing it.
—*Oscar Hammerstein II*

The advancement of nursing interventions and knowledge of effective nursing protocols to achieve optimal outcomes has exploded in the last decade. Awareness of evidence to support nursing practice has not grown as rapidly as the valuable resources that are available. Educating nurses to achieve optimal outcomes based on the best evidence available is among the greatest challenges that emerge in the health care environment mandated to change. The profession of nursing is indebted to organizations such as the Robert Wood Foundation that not only supports the development of research for use in practice but also provides support for the translation of research into practice. For, what good is the best evidence if it does not transition into practice, or is not effectively utilized? What good is the most beautiful sounding bell, if not rung, or the most endearing song, if not sung?

One state program that has embraced the challenge is the Hawaii State Center for Nursing's innovative statewide Evidence-based Practice Program. Initiatives such as these serve as models for other states and regions in the development of programs to transition evidence into practice. The most valuable evidence in effecting optimal patient outcomes is only as viable as those who understand the evidence and its value and can transition this knowledge into practice.

Instituting evidence- based practice is not just about the research that is available. It incorporates the nurse's personal knowledge and experience, patient preferences, available resources, and the best research information.[1] Nursing leaders assume much responsibility in assuring that evidence is used in practice, which goes far

Nurs Clin N Am 49 (2014) xiii–xiv
http://dx.doi.org/10.1016/j.cnur.2014.07.001
0029-6465/14/$ – see front matter © 2014 Elsevier Inc. All rights reserved.

beyond basic nursing interventions and incorporates several major steps. These steps are simple, but critical for appropriate utilization of evidence. Nurses at all levels are charged with asking questions that are germane and answerable, accessing the best information, evaluating the information for validity and significance, applying the information to patient care, and evaluating the impact of the evidence in relation to expected outcomes.[1] This does not happen without an organized and concerted effort among all of those involved in patient care.

There are many popular terms in nursing that seem to come and go. Many in our profession are continually perplexed as to whether the recipients of nursing care are "clients" or "patients." In some nursing curricula, one will see "Med-Surg Nursing" as an area in of study, whereas other curricula will identify "Adult Health Nursing" as an area of study. Although the terms change, the essence of our practice does not. "Evidence-based Practice" is much more than a term, it is a process. It is a process of meaningful use of many elements afforded nurses to effect what is currently the best care available to our clients, or is it "patients?"

Stephen D. Krau, PhD, RN, CNE
Vanderbilt University Medical Center School of Nursing
461 21st Avenue South
Nashville, TN 37240, USA

E-mail address:
steve.krau@vanderbilt.edu

REFERENCE

1. Gillam S, Siriwardena AN. Evidenced-based healthcare and quality improvement. Qual Prim Care 2014;22(3):125–32.

Preface

Empowering Nurses to Utilize Evidence for Better Patient Care

In pockets across the United States, nurse leaders test innovations to improve care in hospitals, community settings, and the home. Nurses, for example, may develop a detailed care plan with hospitalized patients and their families to help them transition to their home or community-based care. A clinical nurse leader may be tasked with care coordination and chronic care management on a hospital floor. In other hospitals throughout the country, staff nurses who participated in the Robert Wood Johnson Foundation–funded *Transforming Care at the Bedside* program continue to suggest changes that they think will improve patient care. The changes are tested over a short period and are adopted if they are proven beneficial. This program has improved patient outcomes and given participating nurses leadership skills.

Nurses, who make up the largest segment of the health care workforce and spend the most time with patients and their families, are crucial to addressing the many challenges facing our health and health care system: an aging and sicker population, millions more insured, a primary care provider shortage, lack of preventive care, and skyrocketing costs. The Institute of Medicine (IOM) recognized the potential for the nursing field to transform health and health care in *The Future of Nursing: Leading Change, Advancing Health,* a report that called on the nursing field to be prepared for health system transformation—and stated that nurses must help to lead and shape this change (IOM. The Future of Nursing: Leading Change, Advancing Health. Washington, DC: The National Academies Press; 2011). The Robert Wood Johnson Foundation and the AARP believed that these recommendations in this report could drastically improve health and health care, so we launched the *Future of Nursing: Campaign for Action*, a 50-state initiative to implement the recommendations. Nurse leaders and their business, philanthropic, consumer, health professional, insurance, and hospital and health system partners are working to promote nursing leadership, practice, and education. Our health care system needs nurses to actively innovate to improve patient care and it is vital for nurses to employ the best available evidence to ensure that their innovations are, in fact, improving patient care. The landmark IOM report, *Crossing the Quality Chasm,* definitively stated that health professionals and policymakers must employ evidence-based practice (EBP) to close the quality chasm (IOM, 2001). EBP enables nurses to use scientifically proven evidence for delivering high-quality patient care.

One of the challenges, however, is that few nurses are trained in EBP. That is why the Hawaii State Center for Nursing's innovative statewide EBP program, consisting of an annual workshop followed by an 18-month internship program, offers a promising model of how to successfully use multidisciplinary teams to spread EBP across health care settings. The Hawaii State Center for Nursing program involves 15 health care organizations and 58 evidence-based projects. Projects have ranged from identifying EBPs to minimize fever to prevent secondary brain injury in the neuroscience patient

Nurs Clin N Am 49 (2014) xv–xvi
http://dx.doi.org/10.1016/j.cnur.2014.05.014
0029-6465/14/$ – see front matter © 2014 Published by Elsevier Inc.

nursing.theclinics.com

population to using EBPs to reduce respiratory complications and intensive care unit length of stay in patients with acute cervical spinal cord injuries. In addition to improving care, this program has equipped participating nurses with the requisite leadership skills to advance in their careers. The program is advancing the IOM goals of strengthening nursing education, practice, and leadership to improve patient care.

This issue begins with an overview that distinguishes EBP and translation science, followed by a description of Hawaii's statewide EBP program that uses active and multifaceted translation science strategies to facilitate the rate and extent of adoption of EBP changes. With one exception, the remaining articles describe individual EBP projects from five different health care facilities that used the Iowa Model to guide their work. Each article includes an evidence summary, a description of implementation strategies, an evaluation of the innovation, and lessons learned. These completed projects were initiated between 2009 and 2012, address a variety of topical nursing issues, and, for the most part, focus on preventing complications (ie, blood sugar elevations, increased lengths of stay, extubation failures, noise-related injury, pain, surgical site infections, pneumonia, restraint use, delirium, and fever). An additional article describes the use of evidence to inform simulation-based learning, a possible strategy for ensuring competencies in and compliance with EBP interventions.

It is my hope that nursing leaders in other states will read this issue of *Nursing Clinics of North America* and seriously consider replicating Hawaii's program to engage nurses in EBP to improve patient care. The Hawaii program demonstrates that health care quality can be realized by employing the best available evidence and empowering the nursing workforce. It also offers a glimpse of the care that the future nursing workforce could provide to create a health system that provides accessible, affordable and quality care to everyone in the United States.

Susan B. Hassmiller, PhD, RN, FAAN
Robert Wood Johnson Foundation
Route 1 and College Road East
PO Box 2316
Princeton, NJ 08543-2316, USA

E-mail address:
SHASSMILLER@rwjf.org

Overview of Evidence-based Practice and Translation Science

Marita G. Titler, PhD, RN

KEYWORDS

- Evidence-based practice • Translation science • National Nursing Practice Network
- Patient outcomes

KEY POINTS

- Evidence-based practice and translation science are not interchangeable terms.
- An emerging body of knowledge in translation science provides an empirical base on effective implementation strategies to promote adoption of evidence-based practices in real world settings.
- The Hawaii State Center for Nursing is at the forefront of providing professional development opportunities that enable nurses to lead EBP programs and projects to improve health and health care.

The application of evidence to improve quality of care and patient outcomes is central to health care improvement. Several Institute of Medicine (IOM) reports describe multiple opportunities for implementation of evidence in health care to improve population health and health care delivery.[1–5] For example, the Clinical and Translational Science Award (CTSA) program of the National Institutes of Health (NIH), by definition, focuses on clinical and translational research, including translation of clinical trial results and other research findings, into practices and communities.[6] The 61 funded CTSAs are expected to partner with communities, practices, and clinicians in not only setting strategic directions for research but also in translating findings from research into health and health care.[6]

EVIDENCE-BASED PRACTICE AND TRANSLATION SCIENCE

Evidence-based practice (EBP) is the conscientious and judicious use of current best evidence in conjunction with clinical expertise and patient values to guide health care

Funding Sources: Dr M.G. Titler: Michigan Institute for Clinical and Health Research. (MICHR) Grant number: 2UL1TR000433.

Division Chair Health Systems Leadership and Effectiveness Science, University of Michigan School of Nursing, UMHS, 400 North Ingalls, Suite 4170, Ann Arbor, MI 48109-5482, USA

E-mail address: mtitler@umich.edu

decisions.[7–10] Best evidence includes findings from randomized controlled trials, evidence from other scientific methods such as descriptive and qualitative research, as well as information from case reports and scientific principles. In contrast, translation science is a field of research that focuses on testing implementation interventions to improve uptake and use of evidence to improve patient outcomes and population health, and to explicate what implementation strategies work for whom, in what settings, and why.[11–13] An emerging body of knowledge in translation science provides an empirical base for guiding the selection of implementation strategies to promote adoption of EBPs in real-world settings.[12,14–24] Thus, EBP and translation science, although related, are not interchangeable terms; EBP is the application of evidence in practice (the doing of EBP), whereas translation science is the study of implementation interventions, factors, and contextual variables that affect knowledge uptake and use in practices and communities.

An important guiding principle for promoting adoption of EBPs is that the attributes of the evidence-based topic (eg, temperature regulation in neurology care) as perceived by users and stakeholders, such as ease of use and strength of the evidence, are neither stable features nor sure determinants of their adoption. It is the interaction among the characteristics of the evidence-base of the topic (eg, specificity, clarity), the intended users (physicians, nurses, pharmacists), and a particular context of practice (eg, inpatient, ambulatory, long-term care setting) that determines the extent of adoption of the EBP.[18] Promoting use of evidence in practice is an active process that is facilitated, in part, by localization of the evidence for use in a specific health care setting, setting forth clear EBP recommendations (eg, practice standard), use of opinion leaders and change champions to promote adoption, modeling and imitation of others who have successfully adopted the EBP, and an organizational culture that values and supports use of evidence to guide practice.[18,25–27] Many of these strategies were used by the nurses who describe their EBP projects in this issue.

Several conceptual models have been tested and are used to guide implementation of evidence-based practice recommendations.[13,15,24,28–31] Common among these models are syntheses of the evidence and setting forth EBP recommendations, implementation of the EBPs, evaluation of the impact on patient care, and consideration of the context/setting in which the evidence is implemented. The Iowa Model of EBP to Promote Quality Care is a practice model designed to guide clinicians in selecting practice topics amenable to EBP, and to implement those practices to improve quality of care.[32] This model, widely used throughout the United States and abroad, is the model that guided nurses in leading the EBP projects described in this issue.

THE NATIONAL NURSING PRACTICE NETWORK

The National Nursing Practice Network (NNPN), established in 2005, provides members of participating health care organizations with access to resources, online learning, and interactive education on EBP. It is a collaborative learning network in which clinicians from participating organizations share their expertise in leading interdisciplinary health care teams in application of evidence in practice through an interactive Web site (www.nnpnetwork.org), webinars, and workgroups.[33] For example, the NNPN hosts a webinar each month to discuss a research article using a journal club format, or to learn about the evidence base of a clinical topic from an expert. Presentations are videotaped for future use. Other resources include podcasts on a variety of EBP topics, guides for critique of research, and Eyes on Evidence documents that summarize practice recommendations. Nurses who lead and contribute to EBP in their organization, and specific EBP projects, are featured on the NNPN Web site to share with others what they are doing and the lessons learned from this work. There are about 1600 to 2000 visits to the NNPN Web site each month. Webinar participants provide valuable feedback about future topics and give examples of how they use the information in their practice.

At present, the NNPN is composed of 107 hospitals and health systems across the United States representing 32 states. It is supported, in part, by the University of Michigan CTSA, and the School of Nursing. The use of a collaborative nursing network provides an innovative way to address challenges in implementing and sustaining EBP in organizations and to maximize sharing of resources and knowledge. It also provides a resource for conducting multisite translation science and a venue for large scale-up of EBP projects with other health systems.

NURSING LEADERSHIP IN EBP AND TRANSLATION SCIENCE

Nursing has a rich history of using research in practice, pioneered by Florence Nightingale who used data to change practices that contributed to high mortality in hospitals and communities.[34–37] Although during the early and mid 1900s few nurses built on the solid foundation of research use exemplified by Nightingale,[38] more recently the nursing profession has provided major leadership for improving care through application of research findings in practice.[39] Nurses are now leading the way in translation science[24,40,41] and EBP[42–46] and, as a result, the scientific body of knowledge translation and the application of evidence in health care are growing.

Nursing brings a steadfast commitment to improved safety, quality of care, and fostering improved patient outcomes. As noted in the IOM report on the future of nursing,[47] nursing associations and the profession are called to provide professional development opportunities that enable nurses to lead programs and projects to improve health and health care. The Hawaii State Center for Nursing is at the forefront of meeting this recommendation through their Evidence-Based Practice and Internship Program to develop a workforce of nurses with competencies in EBP and to improve the quality of health care for their citizens. The articles in this issue will help others understand the process of applying evidence in practice to improve care for a variety of topics using the lessons learned from this work.

We challenge nurses and other state centers for nursing to make a similar commitment to improving care in their states. This is a challenge but also an important opportunity for nurses to lead interdisciplinary health care teams in understanding the importance of EBP and the process of improving quality of care through application of evidence at the point of care delivery. The Hawaii State Center for Nursing, in collaboration with nursing leaders throughout the state, have set in motion an infrastructure and process to address quality of care for multiple populations and types of health care practices in Hawaii. Lessons learned from this approach offer valuable information for others in the United States.

SUMMARY

EBP and translation science are different terms with different processes. The articles in this special issue focus on EBPs for a variety of topics with many lessons to share about the challenges and opportunities in aligning clinician practice behaviors with the evidence. The infrastructure and commitment from the Hawaii State Center for Nursing and nurse leaders in Hawaii is an important model for others to use in maximizing the leadership, strength, and knowledge of nurses in improving quality of care through application of evidence in health care.

REFERENCES

1. IOM (Institute of Medicine). Initial national priorities for comparative effectiveness research. Washington, DC: Institute of Medicine (IOM); 2009.
2. IOM (Institute of Medicine). Clinical practice guidelines we can trust. Washington, DC: Institute of Medicine (IOM); 2011.
3. IOM (Institute of Medicine). For the public's health; investing in a healthier future. Washington, DC: Institute of Medicine (IOM); 2012.
4. IOM (Institute of Medicine). Establishing transdisciplinary professionalism for improving health outcomes: workshop summary. Washington, DC: Institute of Medicine (IOM); 2013.
5. IOM (Institute of Medicine). Core measurement needs for better care, better health, and lower costs: counting what counts: workshop summary. Washington, DC: Institute of Medicine (IOM); 2013.
6. IOM (Institute of Medicine). The CTSA program at NIH: opportunities for advancing clinical and translational research. Washington, DC: Institute of Medicine (IOM); 2013.
7. Cook D. Evidence-based critical care medicine: a potential tool for change. New Horiz 1998;6(1):20–5.
8. Jennings BM, Loan LA. Misconceptions among nurses about evidence-based practice. J Nurs Scholarsh 2001;33(2):121–7.
9. Sackett DL, Straus SE, Richardson WS, et al. Evidence-based medicine: how to practice and teach EBM. London: Churchill Livingstone; 2000.
10. Titler MG, Adam S. Developing an evidence-based practice. In: LoBiondo-Wood G, Haber J, editors. Nurs res. 6th edition. St Louis (MO): Mosby-Year Book; 2006. p. 385–437.
11. Eccles MP, Mittman BS. Welcome to implementation science. Implement Sci 2006;1(1):1.
12. Titler MG. Translation science and context. Res Theory Nurs Pract 2010;24(1):35.
13. Titler MG, Everett LQ. Translating research into practice. Considerations for critical care investigators. Crit Care Nurs Clin North Am 2001;13(4):587–604.
14. Brooks JM, Titler MG, Ardery G, et al. Effect of evidence-based acute pain management practices on inpatient costs. Health Serv Res 2009;44(1):245–63. http://dx.doi.org/10.1111/j.1475-6773.2008.00912.x.
15. Dobbins M, Hanna SE, Ciliska D, et al. A randomized controlled trial evaluating the impact of knowledge translation and exchange strategies. Implement Sci 2009;4(1):61.
16. Feldman PH, Murtaugh CM, Pezzin LE, et al. Just-in-time evidence-based e-mail "reminders" in home health care: impact on patient outcomes. Health Serv Res 2005;40(3):865.
17. Flodgren G, Parmelli E, Doumit G, et al. Local opinion leaders: effects on professional practice and health care outcomes. Cochrane Database Syst Rev 2011;(8):CD000125. http://dx.doi.org/10.1002/14651858.CD000125.pub4.
18. Greenhalgh T, Robert G, Bate P, et al. Diffusion of innovations in health service organisations: a systematic literature review. Malden (MA): Blackwell Publishing; 2005.
19. Hysong SJ, Best RG, Pugh JA. Audit and feedback and clinical practice guideline adherence: making feedback actionable. Implement Sci 2006;1:9. http://dx.doi.org/10.1186/1748-5908-1-9.
20. Ivers N, Jamtvedt G, Flottorp S, et al. Audit and feedback: effects on professional practice and healthcare outcomes. Cochrane Database Syst Rev 2012;6(6):CD000259.

21. Jordan ME, Lanham HJ, Crabtree BF, et al. The role of conversation in health care interventions: enabling sensemaking and learning. Implement Sci 2008;4(1):15.
22. McDonald MV, Pezzin LE, Feldman PH, et al. Can just-in-time, evidence-based "reminders" improve pain management among home health care nurses and their patients? J Pain Symptom Manage 2005;29(5):474–88. http://dx.doi.org/10.1016/j.jpainsymman.2004.08.018.
23. Ploeg J, Skelly J, Rowan M, et al. The role of nursing best practice champions in diffusing practice guidelines: a mixed methods study. Worldviews Evid Based Nurs 2010;7(4):238–51. http://dx.doi.org/10.1111/j.1741-6787.2010.00202.x.
24. Titler MG, Herr K, Brooks JM, et al. Translating research into practice intervention improves management of acute pain in older hip fracture patients. Health Serv Res 2009;44(1):264.
25. Berwick DM. Disseminating innovations in health care. JAMA 2003;289(15): 1969–75.
26. Gillbody S, Whitty P, Grimshaw J, et al. Educational and organizational interventions to improve the management of depression in primary care (a systematic review). JAMA 2003;289(23):3145–51.
27. Rogers EM. Diffusion of innovations. 5th edition. New York: The Free Press; 2003.
28. Damschroder LJ, Aron DC, Keith RE, et al. Fostering implementation of health services research findings into practice: a consolidated framework for advancing implementation science. Implement Sci 2008;4(1):50.
29. Davies P, Walker AE, Grimshaw JM. A systematic review of the use of theory in the design of guideline dissemination and implementation strategies and interpretation of the results of rigorous evaluations. Implement Sci 2008;5(1):14.
30. Grol RP, Bosch MC, Hulscher ME, et al. Planning and studying improvement in patient care: the use of theoretical perspectives. Milbank Q 2007;85(1):93.
31. Rycroft-Malone J, Bucknall T. Models and frameworks for implementing evidence-based practice: linking evidence to action. Evidence based nursing series. Chichester (United Kingdom), Ames (IA): Wiley-Blackwell; 2010.
32. Titler MG, Kleiber C, Steelman VJ, et al. The Iowa model of evidence-based practice to promote quality care. Crit Care Nurs Clin North Am 2001;13(4):497–509.
33. Adams S, Titler MG. Building a learning collaborative. Worldviews Evid Based Nurs 2010;7(3):165–73. http://dx.doi.org/10.1111/j.1741-6787.2009.00170.x.
34. Nightingale F. Notes on matters affecting the health, efficiency, and hospital administration of the British Army. London: Harrison and Sons; 1858.
35. Nightingale F. A contribution to the sanitary history of the British Army during the late war with Russia. London: John W Parker and Sons; 1859.
36. Nightingale F. Notes on hospitals. London: Longman, Green, Roberts, Green; 1863.
37. Nightingale F. Observation on the evidence contained in the statistical reports submitted by her to the Royal Commission on the sanitary state of the Army in India. London: Edward Stanford; 1863.
38. Titler MG. Critical analysis of research utilization (RU): an historical perspective. Am J Crit Care 1993;2(3):264.
39. Kirchhoff KT. State of the science of translational research: from demonstration projects to intervention testing. Worldviews Evid Based Nurs 2004;1(S1):S6–12.
40. Estabrooks CA, Derksen L, Winther C, et al. The intellectual structure and substance of the knowledge utilization field: a longitudinal author co-citation analysis, 1945-2004. Implement Sci 2008;3:49.
41. Titler MG. The evidence for evidence-based practice implementation. In: Hughes R, editor. Patient safety and quality: an evidence-based handbook for

nurses. 1st edition. Rockville (MD): Agency for Healthcare Research and Quality (AHRQ); 2008. p. 1–49. Available at: http://www.ahrq.gov/qual/nurseshdbk/.

42. Dickinson S, Shever LL. Evidence-based nursing innovations. Crit Care Nurs Q 2012;35(1):1.

43. Kelley PW. Evidence-based practice in the military healthcare system. Nurs Res 2010;59(1):S1. http://dx.doi.org/10.1097/NNR.0b013e3181c9764d.

44. Madsen D, Sebolt T, Cullen L, et al. Listening to bowel sounds: an evidence-based practice project. Am J Nurs 2005;105(12):40.

45. Shever LL, Dickinson S. Mobility: a successful investment for critically ill patients. Foreword. Crit Care Nurs Q 2013;36(1):1.

46. Titler MG. Nursing science and evidence-based practice. West J Nurs Res 2011; 33(3):291–5. http://dx.doi.org/10.1177/0193945910388984.

47. IOM (Institute of Medicine). The future of nursing: leading change, advancing health. Washington, DC: Institute of Medicine (IOM); 2011.

Hawaii's Statewide Evidence-based Practice Program

Debra D. Mark, PhD, RN[a],*, Rene'e W. Latimer, MPH, MSN, RN[b],
Joan P. White, MBA, RN[c], Deborah Bransford, BSN, RN, CDE[d],
Katherine G. Johnson, MS, RN, APRN, CCRN, CNRN, CNS-BC[d],
Valerie L. Song, BA[c]

KEYWORDS

- Evidence-based practice program • Nursing • Diffusion of innovations
- Translation science • Implementation science

KEY POINTS

- Hawaii's innovative statewide evidence-based practice (EBP) program, consisting of an annual workshop followed by an 18-month internship program, facilitates practice change across multiple healthcare systems.
- Hawaii's EBP program is generally and positively transforming health care by empowering nurses with the skills and knowledge needed to effectively change practice. However, it cannot be assumed that the consequences of an innovation will always be positive.
- The importance of measuring the impact of EBP cannot be overstated given the resources required.

INTRODUCTION

In the United States, the Patient Protection and Affordable Care Act (2010)[1] and the Institute of Medicine's (IOM) Initiative on the Future of Nursing highlight the ability of nursing to affect the transformation of health care. The IOM defines a model system as "*seamless, affordable, quality care that is accessible to all, patient centered, and*

Funding: This project was partially funded by the Agency for Healthcare Research & Quality, 5R13HS017892 and the Hawaii State Center for Nursing.
[a] Hawai'i State Center for Nursing, University of Hawai'i School of Nursing & Dental Hygiene, 2528 McCarthy Mall, Webster Hall 402, Honolulu, HI 96822, USA; [b] Queen Emma Nursing Institute, The Queen's Medical Center, 1301 Punchbowl Street, Honolulu, HI 96813-2499, USA; [c] Hawai'i State Center for Nursing, 2528 McCarthy Mall, Webster Hall 402, Honolulu, HI 96822, USA; [d] The Queen's Medical Center, 1301 Punchbowl Street, Honolulu, HI 96813-2499, USA
* Corresponding author.
E-mail address: debramar@hawaii.edu

evidence based and leads to improved health outcomes" (IOM, 2011, p. 1).[2] However, delays in translating research into practice continue to impede progress toward attaining this goal.[3–7] The Hawai'i State Center for Nursing (the Center), established in 2003,[8] has a legislative mandate to "conduct research on best practice and quality outcomes" and, more importantly, a vested interest in supporting nurses in their efforts to provide the highest possible quality of care to the people of Hawaii. Efforts in Hawaii to promote use of evidence-based nursing care face typical issues of integrating evidence into practice, but are particularly challenged by island geography and the remote location of practice sites. As a result, the Center took the lead and partnered with facilities across the state to develop an evidence-based practice (EBP) program with the dual purpose of developing an EBP-competent nursing workforce and improving the quality of nursing care to Hawaii's citizens.

EVIDENCE FOR PRACTICE IMPROVEMENT

Many nurses are aware of the importance of EBP, but often do not have the skills, support, or resources to change practice accordingly. Assumptions and misconceptions about EBP are common and few practicing nurses and nurse leaders have received training in EBP. Instead, research findings are used haphazardly and considerable variability in practice patterns results, potentially leading to adverse patient outcomes. Knowing the importance of EBP is not enough; nurses must have the requisite skills and knowledge to translate research findings into practice using the principles of translation science.

Translation science is defined as the study of interventions and variables that influence the rate of adoption of an innovation.[7] Translation science is based on the seminal works of Rogers[6] (2003), who defined the primary characteristics that affect the rate and extent of adoption of an innovation as: (1) characteristics of the innovation; (2) communication processes; (3) social systems; and (4) users of the innovation.[6,9]

The translation science literature has outlined key elements of a successful EBP culture and indicates that multifaceted active dissemination strategies are needed to promote the use of research evidence in clinical and administrative health care decision making. These strategies need to address both the individual practitioner and the organizational perspective, such as the use of mentors, collaborative partnering, EBP champions, time, resources, and administrative support.[4–7,10–14] This article describes and evaluates the implementation strategies of Hawaii's statewide EBP program using Rogers'[6] Diffusion of Innovation (2003) framework and concludes with lessons learned and recommendations.

IMPLEMENTATION STRATEGIES
The Innovation

An innovation is defined as an idea or practice that is perceived as new by users. Hawaii's EBP program is innovative in its statewide approach, encouraging incorporation of EBPs across multiple health care social systems by many users. The current program involves 15 health care organizations and 58 different EBP projects, and consists of an annual workshop followed by an 18-month internship program.

Annual workshop

The Center offers 35 participants an annual 2.5-day workshop that comprises each step of the Iowa Model, which was developed by Dr Marita Titler.[15] The steps are (1) identify triggers, (2) form a team, (3) assemble and critique the literature, (4) synthesize the literature, (5) pilot the practice change, (6) implement the practice change, and (7) evaluate the practice change.

The agenda consists of the Iowa Model didactic steps, followed by activities and exemplars that offer insight into the EBP process. The exemplars are presented by team members from prior classes who describe their project experience while emphasizing a particular phase of the Iowa Model; they also discuss challenges and their efforts at problem solving.

When possible, attendees form teams consisting of a staff nurse, an advanced practice registered nurse (APRN), and a nurse manager. Within this format, the staff nurse serves as a change champion; the APRN acts as an opinion leader, assisting with identifying and critiquing literature and developing implementation strategies; and the nurse manager provides administrative and logistical support. Before the workshop, teams submit a clinical question or problem statement that serves as the foundation for the workshop and internship activities.

Internship program

Although all facets of the Iowa Model are covered during the workshop, a thorough understanding of the model is difficult to convey within the time allotted, and a companion internship program deconstructs each phase into manageable steps. The 18-month internship program is structured around bimonthly meetings that provide 4 hours of interactive didactic content that reinforces workshop material, followed by teams sharing status reports and actions to resolve problems (**Table 1**).

In addition to the Iowa Model reinforcement, content is provided during the internship program that generally coincides with the needs of the teams at that time. For example, sessions may be offered that assist with: (1) reviewing and reworking the PICO (Patient, Intervention, Comparison, Outcome) statement; (2) briefing leadership; (3) searching the literature; (4) literature critique practice sessions; (5) distinguishing process improvement, EBP, and research; (6) submitting to institutional review boards; (7) creating data displays; (8) writing an abstract; (9) preparing a podium or poster presentation; (10) writing guidelines and policies; and (11) writing a project summary.

Curricular revisions

Evaluations are used to modify the curriculum in an effort to improve achievement of learner objectives and competencies. Now in its fifth year, the EBP workshop has been revised annually, but remains at 2.5 days and has continued to follow the steps of the Iowa Model. Revisions are based on formal evaluations completed by the participants and informal evaluations in the form of feedback solicited from each site's EBP coordinator over the course of the subsequent 18-month internship. Dr Titler's continued participation in the workshop has been essential because she brings a wealth of experience to the teams and faculty that cannot easily be reproduced by other faculty members.

Attributes or Characteristics of the Innovation

Characteristics of an innovation that affect the rate and extent of adoption include its relative advantage, compatibility, complexity, ability to be trialed, and observability.[6]

Relative advantage

The Center's central role in the community places it in the position to lead this initiative by bringing together previously fragmented programs and providing the advantage of shared resources in terms of education, expertise, and personnel. The EBP program is supported by several fiscal sources: (1) a 3-year conference grant, funded by the Agency for Healthcare Research and Quality (5R13HS017892), supports the annual

Table 1
Internship program curriculum

MTG	Teams	Phases of Iowa Model and Other Agenda Items	MTG	Teams	Phases of Iowa Model and Other Agenda Items
#1	Current	Phase 1: identify topic and forming a team 1. Following the Iowa Model 2. Identification of triggers 3. Determining organizational priorities 4. PICO	#6	Current	Phase 5: piloting the project 1. Design, implement, evaluate pilot 2. Determining data collection strategy 3. Monitoring the structure, process, and outcome data 4. Data analysis and data displays
	ALL Ongoing	5. Progress reports 6. Individual teams work w/faculty or on projects 7. Writing a policy and guideline 8. Writing an article for publication		ALL Ongoing	5. Progress reports 6. Teams work on refining/rehearsing PIN presentations 7. Writing a policy and guideline 8. Writing an article for publication
#2	Current	Phases 2 and 3: form a team and assemble the literature 1. Forming and managing a team 2. Finding and accessing the literature 3. Reading the literature 4. Critiquing formats 5. Critiquing a guideline/research article 6. Using Excel spreadsheets	#7	Current	Phase 6: instituting EBP changes 1. Assessing team, unit, and organizational readiness 2. Steps needed to institutionalize
	ALL Ongoing	7. Progress reports 8. Ongoing teamwork w/faculty or on projects 9. Writing a policy and guideline 10. Writing an article for publication		ALL Ongoing	3. Progress reports 4. Ongoing teamwork w/faculty or on projects 5. Writing a policy and guideline 6. Writing an article for publication
#3	Current	Phase 4: critique and synthesize the literature 1. Differentiating policy vs guidelines 2. Synthesizing the literature 3. Determining the evidence 4. Presenting findings to leaders	#8	Current	Phase 7: evaluating change 1. Monitoring the change in practice 2. Indicators of adherence 3. Identifying roadblocks to institutionalization
	ALL Ongoing	5. Progress reports 6. Ongoing teamwork w/faculty or on projects 7. Writing a policy and guideline 8. Writing an article for publication		ALL Ongoing	4. Progress reports 5. Ongoing teamwork w/faculty or on projects 6. Writing a policy and guideline 7. Writing an article for publication

(continued on next page)

Table 1 **(continued)**					
MTG	**Teams**	**Phases of Iowa Model and Other Agenda Items**	**MTG**	**Teams**	**Phases of Iowa Model and Other Agenda Items**
#4	Current	Preparing for PIN conference 1. Writing/submitting an abstract to PIN	#9	Current	Summary (red) reports 1. Writing the summary report 2. Enculturating the change
	ALL Ongoing	2. Progress reports 3. Teams work on preparing an abstract 4. Writing a policy and guideline 5. Writing an article for publication		ALL Ongoing	3. Adopting the changes institutionally 4. Write and submit the summary report 5. Progress reports 6. Ongoing teamwork w/faculty or on projects 7. Writing a policy and guideline 8. Writing an article for publication
#5	Current	Developing your presentation for PIN 1. Distinguishing research, PI and EBP 2. Submitting your project to an IRB 3. How to prepare a poster or podium presentation	#10	Current	Next steps 1. Publishing your results 2. Identifying next steps 3. Graduation ceremony
	ALL Ongoing	4. Progress reports 5. Teams work on PIN Presentations 6. Writing a policy and guideline 7. Writing an article for publication		ALL Ongoing	4. Progress reports 5. Ongoing teamwork w/faculty or on projects 6. Writing a policy and guideline 7. Writing an article for publication

Abbreviations: ALL, all team members; MTG, meeting; PIN, pacific institute of nursing conference; w/, with.

EBP workshop; (2) funding for the Project Coordinator; and (3) workshop registration fees of $900 per person. The Center's affiliation with the University of Hawaii gives access to (1) a nursing faculty member who directs the program; (2) statisticians, and (3) medical librarians.

Compatibility
The EBP education program is compatible with the values, experiences, and needs of the community[6] and is well matched with the current drivers of quality health care and patient safety. The program design is similar to other educational programs, inclusive of didactic content and skill development.

Complexity
Simple ideas are adopted more quickly[6] and, at the program level, the Center's EBP approach, which consists of 3 basic elements (education, facilitation, and resources), has been perceived as straightforward and easy to understand. The use of a conceptual model assists in decreasing the complexity of the innovation. The Center, along

with support from community partners, chose the Iowa Model[15] for several reasons: (1) a relationship between Hawai'i facilities and Dr Titler had been established and was long-standing; (2) Dr Titler was willing and available to provide support; (3) the Iowa Model was already in use at one of the major medical centers in Hawaii, and (4) the Iowa Model uses a nonlinear but logical sequence, is organizationally sensitive, and uses all types of evidence to guide practice. Implementation of each project at the unit level, and individual institutions and the Center, work together to diminish the complexity[16] and remove barriers using additional education, resources, consultation, and support, as needed.

Ability to be trialed

The ability to trial an innovation also enhances the rate and extent of innovation adoption. The program was piloted at a major medical center in Hawaii for 2 years; this pilot served as the basis for the Center's program. Modeled after the Advanced Practice Institute at the University of Iowa and facilitated by Dr Marita Titler, the pilot included an initial workshop, an 18-month internship program facilitation by a nursing research office, and grant resources.[12] Also, the use of a conceptual model (the Iowa Model) allows a step-by-step approach to implementation.[15]

Observability

Several teams have successfully disseminated their project results and promoted the observability of the program through national and local podium and poster presentations, Center newsletter and electronic publications, and textbooks.[17] Briefings about the program are also provided to nursing leaders, professional organizations, health care organizations, and the state legislature.

Although the impetus for quality of care and EBP is strong across the health care spectrum in Hawaii, financial constraints and competing priorities limit some organizations' ability to realize the relative advantage of the program. Tertiary care organizations consistently join in program activities, but smaller institutions often lack the resources to participate fully.

Communication Channels or Processes

According to Rogers[6] (2003), communication is "the process by which participants create and share information with one another in order to reach a mutual understanding" (p. 18). Communication is generally categorized into interpersonal and mass media channels, and Hawaii's EBP program uses an array of mechanisms to disseminate information about EBP throughout the state.

Interpersonal channels

The Center uses regularly scheduled meetings as the main venue for interpersonal communication. In addition to the bimonthly internship program sessions, the Center established a steering committee composed of local nursing leaders and EBP experts to facilitate implementation of the EBP program across the state. The steering committee consists of community representatives from various health care institutions including long-term and home care facilities and meets bimonthly (preceding the internship program) to (1) review/refine the strategic plan; (2) assist with problem resolution; (3) provide liaison with the community at large; and (4) review the teams' progress reports.

Mass media channels

The use of mass media also plays an important role in communication, and a group Listserv is maintained by the Center. In addition, the Center's Web site contains a description of the program that is available to the public with exclusive content for

EBP team members and their Chief Nurse Executives (CNEs) that can be accessed via a password-protected link that directs them to summary reports, PowerPoint presentations, templates, and other EBP resources. The Center also capitalizes on Nurses' Week and other special events and uses public radio, television, and print media to promote awareness about nursing and EBP.

Social Systems

Rogers[6] (2003) defines a social system as a set of interrelated units that are engaged in joint problem solving to accomplish a common goal and that affects the innovation's diffusion in several ways: (1) through a communication structure; (2) based on a foundation of system norms; (3) the use of change champions and opinion leaders who are able to influence other individuals' attitudes or overt behavior informally in a desired way with relative frequency; and (4) with the recognition that there are consequences of innovation: desirable versus undesirable, direct versus indirect, anticipated versus unanticipated.

Communication structure

The communication structure for the statewide initiative was instituted over time as the network of participating institutions expanded. Designated nursing leaders at each health care facility communicate directly with the Center and disseminate EBP information.

Team progress reports are updated every other month and are based on the progress reports discussed at the bimonthly internship program. Once the steering committee reviews the updated progress reports, they are distributed to the team members, posted on our Web site, and shared with the CNE and chief executive officers (CEO) of the participating organizations (**Fig. 1**). The purpose for this report distribution is to increase CNE and CEO awareness of team progress, engender support if a team may be stalled, and track each facility's teams' progress, which may serve to encourage healthy competition across sites or units.

FACILITY	IDENTIFY & PRIORITIZE TOPICS	FORM TEAM	FIND & CRITIQUE LITERATURE	DETERMINE EVIDENCE	PILOT CHANGE	INSTITUTE EBP CHANGES	EVALUATE CHANGE

Fig. 1. Sample progress report.

The Center takes advantage of every opportunity to speak about the EBP program. The Center has made an extra effort to market the EBP program to a variety of health care organizations across the state to encourage participation by their staff and engender support. Briefings have been provided to the local chapter of the American Organization of Nurse Executives; the CEOs of the Healthcare Association of Hawaii, and the Hawaii Association of Directors of Nursing Administration. The state legislature also receives an annual report depicting the outcomes of the EBP program. Also supported by the Agency for Healthcare Research and Quality grant, the annual Pacific Institute of Nursing conference has been an ideal venue for disseminating the products of the EBP projects to other nurses.

System norms

A Center goal is to increase the EBP capacity across the state and engage (1) all health care venues from ambulatory to hospice care; (2) all types of patient and nurse populations; and (3) all types of practice, inclusive of clinical, educational, and administrative practices. The ultimate vision is to institutionalize EBP change. The EBP program's strategic plan is nested under the Center's strategic plan and approved by the Center's advisory board, which sets policy and has representatives from all fields of nursing as well as business, labor, and the community at large.

To ensure commitment and clear articulation of roles, a memorandum of understanding between the Center and each institution delineates expectations for each party (**Box 1**). The Center's responsibilities include offering the annual workshop and internship program, providing support and resources as needed, and procuring grant monies. Teams of nurses, rather than individual nurses, agree to attend the workshop and bimonthly meetings of the internship program, completing the activities of the Iowa Model, joining in dissemination efforts, seeking support as needed, serving as mentors for other nurses interested in EBP, and collaborating across sites where appropriate. Institutions are expected to contribute to the workshop's success by providing paid time and registration fees for participants.

Commitment to the EBP program is also expected by way of leadership support throughout an institution; the importance of this support cannot be overemphasized. A major concern of team members is having available the necessary resources and time to complete an EBP project. Many of the institutions have provided approximately 8 hours per month of paid time to complete the project and this has proved to be a successful strategy.

Opinion leaders and change champions

Since the inception of Hawaii's EBP program, the Center has endorsed the use of opinion leaders who are respected, influential, competent, and passionate about the topic, and change champions who function as informal leaders and expert clinicians committed to quality care. The teams are introduced to these roles and identify the person responsible. In addition, many of the participating institutions have internal opinion leaders who promote EBP while serving on the EBP Steering Committee and as faculty for the program.[18,19]

The Center also supports similar leadership roles to manage the EBP program. The Program Director volunteers as part of his/her university service and provides oversight and direction to the program, functions as a content expert, is knowledgeable about local and national resources available to nurses, and provides support to stalled teams and where resources are minimal. A part-time Project Coordinator works with the Program Director and assists with day-to-day program operations and functions as the point of contact for the community.

Box 1
Memorandum of agreement

The Hawai'i State Center for Nursing (HSCFN) was created and established by the Hawaii State Legislature in 2003. Its purpose is to function as a catalyst to bring varied and diverse organizations together to collaborate on solutions and strategies to address nursing workforce issues. Key areas of emphasis include conducting research on best practices and quality outcomes, recruitment, retention, and nursing workforce data.

The EBP program is a signature initiative of the Center focused on improving the quality of care through advances in care delivery and improved patient outcomes. Nursing staff satisfaction is increased as well. The EBP program accomplishes this by using a structured model that begins with the development of a problem statement and a search of the scientific literature. If sufficient evidence is found to support development of a new or revised intervention, guidelines are developed and the practice change is implemented and evaluated. Nursing care is changed according to current evidence and improvements in quality patient care are realized.

It has been shown that evidence-based patient care has far-reaching positive results that extend through the care delivery system and to the community at large. The Center has made a significant commitment to this program in the forms of staff and budget. The EBP process takes approximately 18 months to complete following an intensive 2.5-day workshop. To be successful, it requires that both parties agree to meet all their commitments throughout the duration of the project.

The following identifies some, although not all, of what the Center and the organization agree to provide over the course of the EBP workshop and internship.

The HSCFN Will:

- Conduct a 2.5-day EBP workshop led by a nationally recognized nursing educator, researcher, and expert in EBP and the creator of the patented Iowa Model for EBP. Lunch or continental breakfast and refreshments will be provided each day.

- Provide expertise in EBP using local research and academic and clinical faculty to continue educating and supporting the teams and projects for the 18-month internship.

- Provide all materials and work books for the workshop and internship.

- Provide assistance with disseminating project findings via poster, podium, and PowerPoint presentations and/or publications.

«ORGANIZATION» will:

- Pay tuition for a team or teams of 2 or 3 members of the organization to attend the 2.5-day workshop.

- Allow the team to participate in the bimonthly all-day internship meetings for a period of 18 months following the workshop.

- Provide leadership, verbal support, and financial and/or other resources necessary to ensure that the project has recognition within the organization and is able to reach completion.

- Assist with drafting or revising policies, procedures, practice protocols, guidelines, and similar institutional documents that will establish the new practice within the organization.

- Foster dissemination beyond the organization by encouraging the team to participate in conferences and other venues that will allow the project to gain widespread recognition and add to the body of evidence-based patient care practices.

- Ensure that the project summary report is completed and sent to HSCFN for dissemination.

- Allow the team to post the summary report of their project on the Center's Web site.

- Ensure that the Project Red Book is completed and readily available within the institution to others as a resource.

- Acknowledge HSCFN's support of the project in their presentations and/or publications.

Consequences of innovation

Rogers[6] (2003) discusses consequences as those changes to individuals and/or social systems that occur as a result of the innovation. Measuring the consequences of the Center's program is a challenge because of the multiple organizations and individuals involved, but markers of success are apparent. The program has affected the professional development of the individual participants. Many have expressed interest in returning to school for graduate work and others have gone on to lead new projects and teams. EBP team leaders are recognized within their institutions for having the requisite leadership skills and are being promoted to positions of increasing authority and responsibility (ie, directors of quality improvement departments). In addition, these individuals have shown an interest in scholarly activities. Dissemination efforts by way of conference presentations, briefings to local stakeholders, and publications are additional skill sets ascribed to the program. Teams have delivered 18 podium and 8 poster presentations at 4 separate local and 2 national conferences. Ten teams are in the process of submitting manuscripts for publication.

Social system change is evident in that one acute care facility hired an EBP mentor to meet with and guide each of the teams toward completion. Another large acute care facility had the resources to hire staff to implement an evidence-based childbirth education course and a discharge planning coordinator.

Users of the Innovation

Rogers[6] (2003) based his categorization of users on the length of time required to adopt an innovation. As seen with any innovation, the acceptance of and participation in the practice change vary among users, and the variation seen in our teams not only correlates with Rogers'[6] categories of adopters (innovators, early adopters, early majority, late majority, or laggards) but with his S-shaped adopter distribution as well.

Users of Hawaii's EBP program include nurses (licensed practical nurses, registered nurses, and APRNs). However, projects typically require multidisciplinary involvement. For example, in a project designed to improve pulmonary management of spinal cord–injured patients, users extended beyond nurses to include physicians, pharmacists, respiratory therapists, rehabilitation therapists, laboratory staff, dietitians, and anesthesia staff. Members of these multidisciplinary teams then became the change champions for EBP in their units and assisted with performance gap assessments; organized focus groups/meetings with staff in their units; completed audits and provided feedback; and piloted, implemented, and evaluated the practice change.

Rogers'[6] adopter categories are typically based on individuals, but may also describe an EBP team and organizational behaviors.[20,21] Just as an innovator or early adopter team can influence a unit to embrace new practice change, a venturesome, respected CNE or CEO can lead an organization to do the same. In addition to the pursuit of high-quality care, organizational drivers for EBP in Hawaii include competition for customers, magnet recertification, contract-driven clinical ladders, and guarding against costs associated with implementation of the Affordable Care Act.[1]

EVALUATION
Rate and Extent of Adoption

The impact of Hawaii's EBP program can be evaluated by the rate and extent of its adoption. The process of adopting an innovation involves sequential stages in which individuals gain knowledge, form an attitude, make a decision, and implement the innovation.[6] This process consists of 5 stages: knowledge, persuasion, decision, implementation, and confirmation.

Knowledge

Exposure to the innovation and gaining an understanding of how it works are the essential elements of the knowledge stage. Competency development in EBP requires knowledge and skills in team leadership, finding and critiquing the literature, developing EBP standards, and implementing and evaluating practice change.[22] Over the past 5 years, 155 nurses representing 15 health care facilities have attended the EBP workshop and have participated, or are participating, in the internship program.

Persuasion

Unlike marketing efforts, persuasion in this case means engagement with the innovation.[6] Although EBP workshop graduates are convinced of the importance of EBP and understand the basic steps of how to begin a project, active involvement in the subsequent internship program is where attitudes toward EBP tend to evolve to a more favorable perspective. The internship offers reinforcement of didactic content and continued support and seems to be a key to successful persuasion.

Decision

Rogers[6] (2003) describes the decision stage as the level at which innovations are adopted or rejected and asserts that trialing an innovation is a precursor to decision making. Hawaii's EBP program uses several mechanisms to facilitate resolution of this stage. First, inherent in the Iowa Model is a pilot phase, in which an EBP project is tested on a small scale before full implementation. Second, exemplars are an integral part of the program, in which previous teams present their projects at the annual workshop and share status reports at each internship meeting. Third, peer pressure is exercised as teams share their successes and challenges with their peers during internship meetings. A tracking mechanism is distributed to individual team members and their immediate and senior leadership (see **Fig. 1**).

Implementation

During the implementation stage, behavior change occurs and may require more time than anticipated.[6] At the program level, the workshop and internship are adjusted based on feedback and evaluations from the EBP teams and the faculty. At the EBP project level, a total of 58 projects have been initiated and, of those, 19 are complete, 12 have been discontinued, and the remaining 27 projects are ongoing and in various stages of the Iowa Model; approximately 30 different patient care topics have been or are being addressed (**Table 2**).

Most teams have required more time than the 18-month internship program to implement their project fully. Problem statements are submitted before the workshop, but over the course of the workshop and into the internship most are reinvented as the teams reevaluate organizational priorities and review the literature. Reinvention may also occur as the innovation is diffused throughout an organization.

Confirmation

Once an innovation decision is made, reinforcement is sought to confirm or reverse it.[6] Most of the projects have been confirmed and implemented across acute care, long-term care, rehabilitation, and psychiatric health care organizations. The sites with the highest rates and extents of adoption are those that have committed leadership and are well resourced.

Facilities with low rates and extent of adoption were challenged to find resources and commitment within their organizations to implement and evaluate their projects successfully. Twelve projects have been discontinued, mainly because of waning organizational support.[20,23]

Table 2
Hawaii's EBP projects: 2009 to 2012

Type of Facility	EBP Topic
Acute care hospital (7)	Accidental extubation in pediatric critical care patients
	Advanced care planning based on cultural beliefs/practices
	Alternative therapy pain management in postoperative joint patients
	Ambient noise levels
	Childbirth education
	Clinical simulation for medication errors in orthopedic/neurologic/vascular units
	Conscious sedation safety
	Culture of transparency to support bedside patient safety
	Decompensation in patients with heart failure
	Early sepsis screening in the emergency room and hospital
	Fall prevention
	Group therapy for adolescents in inpatient psychiatric setting
	Hospital discharge instructions for adults
	Hourly rounding for toileting
	Intraoperative skin preparation for adult hand surgical patients
	Length of stay, negative outcomes, and costs for adults >18 y of age
	Management of sacral pressure ulcers and medication errors in adult surgical patients
	Nonpharmacologic sleep for SICU patients
	Organizational change at the unit level
	Pain management for opioid-dependent orthopedic patients
	Patient choices for coping with labor
	Patient/staff communication
	Perioperative management of adult patients with sleep apnea × 2
	Perioperative hyperglycemia management
	Pulmonary management of patients with spinal cord disorders
	Reduction in hospital-acquired pressure ulcers
	Restraint use reduction in medical/surgical and critical care units
	Restraint use reduction in emergency department
	Shift report process for adult patients
	Simulation training for staff nurses
	Surgical site infections in antepartum/surgical ward
	Trauma informed care
	Vascular access device selection in long-term intravenous patients
Behavioral health hospital	Suicide reduction in inpatient settings
	Restraint use reduction in aggressive behavior children <8 y old
	Aggressive behavior in children <12 y old
	Fall prevention
Critical access hospital	Hospital-acquired infections
Long-term care facility (2)	Pain management for residents with dementia
	Fall prevention × 2
Pediatric hospital	Ventilator weaning readiness
Rehabilitation hospital (2)	Decrease prevention
	Patency of peripheral intravenous lock in children
	Pediatric pin site care in pediatric population w/external fixation
	Postsurgery bowel function
	Surgical/pin wound dressing

Abbreviation: SICU, surgical intensive care unit.

LESSONS LEARNED AND RECOMMENDATIONS FOR OTHERS
Projects Across Institutions and Units

Bimonthly face-to-face meetings have led to a higher level of interinstitutional interaction, but silos still exist. For example, despite having 4 institutions with EBP topics to reduce patient fall rates, it has been difficult to get teams to work together. We anticipated that different teams would want to share literature search strategies and critiquing activities, but, for the most part, each institution seems to prefer to work as a discrete team.

Planned and unplanned multiunit projects were generated at several large acute care facilities. One acute care facility identified restraint reduction as a strategic initiative. Five different units and EBP teams across the facility were selected to develop and implement an organizational EBP standard. The facility found that a standardized approach to restraint reduction on each unit was more challenging than expected because of different patient populations and varying levels of readiness of units to embark on changing the culture of restraint use. However, evidence-based housewide strategies such as data transparency, regular education of staff, and leadership support were effective and have led to an overall reduction in restraint prevalence and hours in restraint. Another team at this same facility initiated a project focused on conscious sedation competency. It was originally intended to affect 1 unit but resulted in a house-wide practice change. Another health care system sent teams from 3 of their 4 acute care hospitals across 2 islands to implement evidence-based, systemwide, advance care planning practices. The 3 teams were challenged with multiple ethnicities, different organizational cultures, and geographic separation; these projects were discontinued.

Organizational Barriers

One challenge has been ensuring that resources are available once nurses engage in EBP. In several facilities, nurses are told that they will be supported for up to 8 hours a month to work on projects. However, this time is not always available and is consistently listed as one of the main barriers to EBP[24,25] even when the time is compensated. Nursing leadership is also challenged by the constraints of time and conflicting priorities, limiting their ability to be vocal, visible champions of EBP and thwarting full integration of the practice change into the organizational culture.[26]

Providing an adequate supply of nursing mentors for EBP projects remains a barrier.[18] About a dozen early workshop participants have gained sufficient mastery of EBP to be able to train others, have taken leadership roles in their institutions, and are teaching and coaching others about EBP. These faculty members are employed by larger health systems that also have a nurse researcher and APRN support through project implementation. The smaller institutions do not have such resources and require more support from the Center.

Measuring financial outcomes in EBP projects has also been difficult. Many of the projects that have been designed and implemented have measured improvements that may lack an obvious economic effect. Proxy measures such as patient satisfaction and length of stay have been used to try to capture financial outcomes, but do not represent the full economic impact.

User Barriers

User barriers may be related to resource gaps, personality variables, and communication behavior.[6] Negative peer opinions and lack of physician reinforcement were some of the barriers that prevented nurses from eagerly adopting a new practice. Multidisciplinary members of our EBP teams also identified the following barriers: differing passion for the practice change, differing priorities for their unit, limited managerial support from their unit, negative impact on workflow, and time needed to support the EBP project.[24]

EBP is a slow process and nurses with previous experience with rapid cycle process improvement projects may struggle with the time it takes to fully review and critique the literature before implementation. EBP is often perceived as a project-based intervention rather than a reasoned and research-informed approach to clinical problem solving and practice improvement. In short, enculturation of EBP has not been fully integrated into the way nurses practice. When asked about EBP in participating institutions, many nurses respond by describing a project on their unit, but may not make the connection to their everyday bedside practice.

Some of the strategies used to overcome these challenges included being receptive to their feedback, sharing the data/outcome measures specific to their unit, embedding the practice change into the electronic medical record (eg, as order sets or to standardize documentation), understanding that using an EBP practice standard is an adjunct to critical thinking, educating all shifts and units involved in the practice change about the reason for the change as well as the EBP process, using algorithms to simplify the practice change, providing easy access to the algorithm and the EBP practice standard, and giving timely feedback on the outcome measures. Projects were best supported when users were identified early in the process and encouraged to provide input into the development of the practice change.

SUMMARY

The Hawai'i State Center for Nursing has a mandate to support nurses in their efforts to provide the highest possible quality of care to the people of Hawaii. The statewide EBP program is one such effort and is generally and positively transforming health care by empowering nurses with the skills and knowledge needed to effectively change practice. However, it cannot be assumed that the consequences of an innovation will always be positive. The importance of measuring the impact of EBP cannot be overstated given the resources required. Successful implementation of innovations tends to be varied and based not only on the evidence but on perceived risk/benefit ratios, concordance with value judgments, confounding variables, and pressures for adoption.[27,28] Explicating the value of this innovation requires continued and thoughtful strategies for evaluation.

ACKNOWLEDGMENTS

Mahalo nui loa to our writing coach, Bee Molina Kooker, DrPH, APRN, NEA-BC, for turning ideas into reality.

REFERENCES

1. Patient Protection and Affordable Care Act of 2010, 42 USC §111–48.
2. Institute of Medicine. The future of nursing: leading change, advancing health. Washington, DC: The National Academies Press; 2011.
3. Cullen L, Titler M, Rempel G. An advanced educational program promoting evidence-based practice. West J Nurs Res 2010;33(3):345–64.
4. Cummings G, Estabrooks C, Midozdzi W, et al. Influence of organizational characteristics and context on research utilization. Nurse Res 2007;56(4):S24–39.

5. McCloskey D. Nurses' perceptions of research utilization in a corporate health care system. J Nurs Scholarsh 2008;40(1):39–45.
6. Rogers E. Diffusion of innovations. New York: Free Press; 2003.
7. Titler M. Translation science and context. Res Theory Nurs Pract 2010;24(1): 35–55.
8. Hawaii HR. 422, Act 198. Relating to a Center for Nursing. 2003.
9. Titler MG, Everett LQ. Translating research into practice: considerations for critical care investigators. Crit Care Nurs Clin North Am 2001;13(4):587–604.
10. Brown D, White J, Leibbrandt L. Collaborative partnerships for nursing faculties and health service providers: what can nursing learn from business literature? J Nurs Manag 2006;14:170–9.
11. Kim S, Brown C, Ecoff L, et al. Regional evidence-based practice fellowship program: impact on evidence-based practice implementation and barriers. Clin Nurs Res 2013;22(1):51–69.
12. Mark DD, Latimer RW, Hardy MD. "Stars" aligned for evidence-based practice: a tri-service initiative in the Pacific. Nurse Res 2010;59(Suppl 1):S48–57.
13. Rutledge D, Donaldson N. Building organizational capacity to engage in research utilization. J Nurs Adm 1995;25(10):12–6.
14. Spoth R, Greenberg M. Impact challenges in community science-with-practice: lessons from PROSPER on transformative practitioner-scientist partnerships and prevention infrastructure development. Am J Community Psychol 2011;48: 106–19.
15. Titler MG, Kleiber C, Steelman VJ, et al. The Iowa model of evidence-based practice to promote quality care. Crit Care Nurs Clin North Am 2001;13(4):497–509.
16. Rycroft-Malone J, Burton C. Paying attention to complexity in implementation research. Worldviews Evid Based Nurs 2010;7(3):121–2. http://dx.doi.org/10.1111/j.1741-6787.2010.00200.x.
17. Melnyk BM. Achieving a high-reliability organization through implementation of the ARCC model for systemwide sustainability of evidence-based practice. Nurs Adm Q 2012;36(2):127–35. http://dx.doi.org/10.1097/naq.0b013e318249fb6a.
18. Lavoie-Tremblay M, Riche MC, Marchionni C, et al. Implementation of evidence-based practices in the context of a redevelopment project in a Canadian health-care organization. J Nurs Scholarsh 2012;44(4):418–27. http://dx.doi.org/10.1111/j.1547-5069.2012.01480.x.
19. Reicherter EA, Gordes KL, Glickman LB, et al. Creating disseminator champions for evidence-based practice in health professions education: an educational case report. Nurse Educ Today 2013;33(7):751–6. http://dx.doi.org/10.1016/j.nedt.2012.12.003.
20. Aarons GA, Sommerfeld DH, Walrath-Greene CM. Evidence-based practice implementation: the impact of public versus private sector organization type on organizational support, provider attitudes, and adoption of evidence-based practice. Implement Sci 2009;4:83. http://dx.doi.org/10.1186/1748-5908-4-83.
21. Green AE, Aarons GA. A comparison of policy and direct practice stakeholder perceptions of factors affecting evidence-based practice implementation using concept mapping. Implement Sci 2011;6:104. http://dx.doi.org/10.1186/1748-5908-6-104.
22. QSEN. QSEN Institute. 2013. Available at: http://qsen.org/about-qsen/. Accessed September 1, 2014.
23. Flodgren G, Rojas-Reyes MX, et al. Effectiveness of organisational infrastructures to promote evidence-based nursing practice. Cochrane Database Syst Rev 2012;(2):CD002212.

24. Chamberlain P, Brown CH, Saldana L. Observational measure of implementation progress in community based settings: the Stages of Implementation Completion (SIC). Implement Sci 2011;6:116. http://dx.doi.org/10.1186/1748-5908-6-116.

25. Melnyk BM, Fineout-Overholt E, Gallagher-Ford L, et al. Sustaining evidence-based practice through organizational policies and an innovative model. Am J Nurs 2011; 111(9):57–60. http://dx.doi.org/10.1097/01.NAJ.0000405063.97774.0e.

26. Sandstrom B, Borglin G, Nilsson R, et al. Promoting the implementation of evidence-based practice: a literature review focusing on the role of nursing leadership. Worldviews Evid Based Nurs 2011;8(4):212–23. http://dx.doi.org/10.1111/j.1741-6787.2011.00216.x.

27. Bick D, Graham I. Evaluating the impact of implementing evidence-based practice. West Sussex (United Kingdom): John Wiley; 2010.

28. Denis J, Hebert Y, Langley A, et al. Explaining diffusion patterns for complex health care innovations. Health Care Manage Rev 2002;27(3):60–73.

Part I: Triggers for an Evidence Based Practice Project

Managing Peri-Operative Hyperglycemia in Total Hip and Total Knee Replacement Surgeries

Maryline Dolor, BSN, RN[a],*, Michele Hadano, MS, RN[a],
Rene'e W. Latimer, MPH, MSN, RN[b]

KEYWORDS

• Hip • Knee • Replacement • Surgery • Surgical Site Infection • Hyperglycemia

KEY POINTS

• Approximately 600,000 total knee arthroplasty (TKA) procedures are performed every year in the United States.

• Examining nursing practice can provide insights into whether practice variation or protocol nonadherence exists. This examination provides an opportunity for descriptive research in the orthopedic setting.

• A descriptive study of risk factors for surgical site infections in patients receiving TKA discovered an infection rate higher than the benchmark.

INTRODUCTION/BACKGROUND

Approximately 600,000 total knee arthroplasty (TKA) procedures are performed every year in the United States (**Fig. 1**). TKA is a costly procedure but results in improved quality of life and functional status and has therefore been deemed highly cost-effective.[1] Since the advent of TKA in early 1991, the volume of these procedures has increased by 161.5% in the US Medicare population. Over the same period, the average length of stay (LOS) for a patient undergoing TKA has decreased from 7.9 days from the period of 1991 to 1994 to 3.5 days in 2007 to 2010.[1]

Disclosures: None.
[a] QET 8DH/Ortho Joint Trauma, The Queen's Medical Center, 1301 Punchbowl Street, Honolulu, HI 96813, USA; [b] Queen Emma Nursing Institute, The Queen's Medical Center, 1301 Punchbowl Street, Honolulu, HI 96813, USA
* Corresponding author.
E-mail address: mdolor@queens.org

Rate per 100 cases

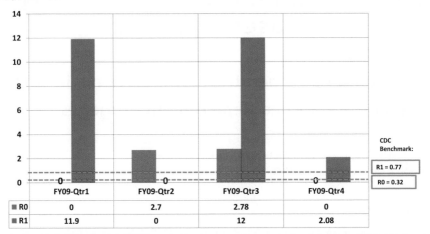

Fig. 1. Surgical site infection (SSI) results for knee replacement for fiscal year 2009. FY, fiscal year.

Surgical site infections (SSIs) are serious operative complications that occur in the surgical site following approximately 2% of surgical procedures and are largely preventable.[2] SSIs in this population decreased from 0.7% to 0.4% in the past 2 decades.[1] Although this reduction in SSIs is laudable, the goal for health care providers is for no TKAs to be complicated by SSIs, because of the burden that they place on patients and hospitals. In a study by Poultsides and colleagues,[3] patients experiencing SSIs after undergoing TKAs had a significantly higher overall comorbidity burden, higher perioperative mortality, longer LOSs, and higher complication rates. The increased burden extends to hospitals as well because the average cost of hospital care was double for patients with SSIs versus patients without SSIs.[2]

Risk factors that have been identified and incorporated into prevention guidelines include preoperative, intraoperative, and postoperative incision care and surveillance (**Table 1**). Despite abundant research examining risk factors for SSIs, there is much less research on strategies to reduce SSIs. Examining nursing practice can provide insights into whether practice variation or protocol nonadherence exists. This examination provides an opportunity for descriptive research in the orthopedic setting. Therefore, this article describes a descriptive research study that was developed from a practice issue that then triggered an evidence-based practice (EBP) project for perioperative hyperglycemia management in knee and hip replacement surgeries.[4]

The focus on perioperative hyperglycemia management in the EBP project after the project described in this article was a result of 2 things: (1) a recognition that there were no practice standards in place for glucose management in this high-risk surgical population, and (2) a growing awareness that the body of evidence for prevention of SSI supported perioperative hyperglycemia management as an important factor for reducing the risk of SSIs.[5]

Setting

This descriptive study took place in an acute-care medical facility accredited by The Joint Commission. The facility is licensed for 505 acute beds and 28 subacute beds and is widely known for its programs in cancer, cardiovascular disease, neuroscience, orthopedics, surgery, emergency medicine and trauma, and behavioral medicine. The

Table 1
SSI risk factors after TKA

Categories	Risk Factors
Patient factors	Age, gender, ethnicity Comorbidities (eg, diabetes, cancer, heart disease) Overweight/obese Current medication (eg, immunosuppression, antihyperglycemics) Preexisting infection Attendance at preoperative class
Procedure factors: preoperative	Standardized preoperative preparation protocol Glucose check
Procedure factors: intraoperative	Skin preparation products Duration of surgery (incision cut to incision close time) Type of wound drain Staff protective gear (space suits) Number of staff in operating room Antibiotic-impregnated cement during procedure Operating room number Certified surgeon
Procedure factors: postoperative	Postoperative day of dressing change Completion of intravenous antibiotics within 24 h after surgery Type of analgesia LOS Date/time to D/C urinary catheter Presence of UTI within 48 h Glucose check Destination at discharge: home, progressive care, SNF
Outcome	Readmission within 30 d for postoperative infection

Abbreviations: D/C, discontinued; SNF, skilled nursing facility; UTI, urinary tract infection.

facility is the only one in the state to have achieved Magnet status (the highest institutional honor for hospital excellence) from the American Nurses Credentialing Center. Magnet recognition is held by less than 6% of hospitals in the United States. Magnet institutions are committed to exemplary nursing practice that must include measurement of quality indicators, use of national benchmarks, data analysis, and performance improvement activities.[6]

Because empirical outcomes are foundational to practice excellence, Magnet organizations seek to incorporate research and evidence into the clinical setting for use by all levels of nurses.[6] This research showed the application of all 4 components of the Magnet model to support bedside nurses in participation in research including: (1) structural empowerment through shared governance and professional development support; (2) transformational leadership through strong nurse manager and director involvement, (3) new knowledge, innovations, and improvements through nursing research department mentorship, and (4) exemplary professional practice through attention to nurse-sensitive indicators (**Table 2**).

EVIDENCE FOR PRACTICE IMPROVEMENT
Identification of the Opportunity

Risk categories for SSIs are based on Centers for Disease Control and Prevention (CDC) criteria including duration of the surgery in terms of cut-point hours, surgical wound classification, and the American Society of Anesthesiologists physical status

Table 2
Operationalizing Magnet components

Magnet Components	Structures and Strategies
(1) Structural empowerment	Shared governance structure: Nursing Products Subcommittee of the Nursing Practice Council Professional development: clinical ladder program that provides resources to support research
(2) Transformational leadership	Strong nurse manager support for research project and development of research nurse Chief nursing officer and director–level support through dedicated resources for proposal development and manuscript preparation
(3) New knowledge, innovations, and improvements	Research fellowship program provides mentored research experience Access to hospital-wide research infrastructure for support, regulatory review, and human subjects review as needed
(4) Exemplary professional practice	Infrastructure to promote EBP Access to hospital-wide quality report card and unit-specific patient care outcomes to monitor progress

Abbreviation: EBP, evidence-based practice.

classification.[7] Risk category 0 means that a patient has no risk factors for developing SSI. Risk category 1 means that a patient has 1 risk factor for developing SSI.

The Nursing Products Subcommittee of the Nursing Practice Council identified a higher-than-national benchmark SSI rate in fiscal year (FY) 2009 (July 2008 to June 2009) among patients receiving TKA (replacement and revision) on a surgical unit in a Magnet facility. The facility's FY 2009 SSI rate for all TKA surgeries was 2.74 per 100 cases (2.16 per 100 cases for risk category 0 and 3.07/100 cases for risk category 1), which is higher than the CDC median benchmark of 0.32 per 100 cases for risk category 0 and 0.77 per 100 cases for risk category 1 (**Fig. 2**). Discussions in the Nursing Products Subcommittee focused on the relationships between SSI and the 2 different surgical preparations being used in the operating room (OR): ChloraPrep and DuraPrep. The current evidence identified 1 preparation as superior

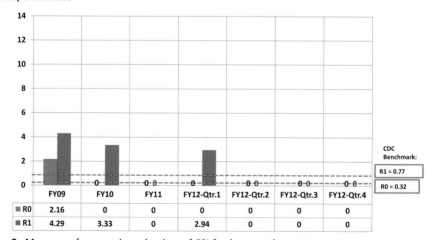

Fig. 2. Measure of success in reduction of SSI for knee replacement.

to others: ChloraPrep.[8–10] Possible practice variations with surgical preparation products were also discussed in relation to SSIs following TKA (see **Fig. 2**).

Methods

An interprofessional team was convened to design and implement a descriptive study to explore evidence-based risk factors for SSI after TKA. The core team consisted of 5 members, including the nurse managers from the OR orthopedic department and from the postoperative in-patient orthopedic unit, the staff research nurse, and representatives from infection prevention and nursing research. The team met monthly to develop the proposal and each member of the team, physicians, infection control personnel, and staff nurses provided a particular perspective during proposal writing and study implementation, which was important for project implementation and development of new practice protocols.

Design

The team determined that current practice on the unit needed to be described before implementing improvement strategies. To that end, a retrospective descriptive study of SSIs in TKA was designed and implemented over a 2-year period, from 2009 to 2011.

Sample

The sample consisted of all patients who had TKA including replacement and revision during the study period. The inclusion criteria were adults 18 years or older who had total knee replacement surgery at the medical center between July 1, 2008, and June 30, 2009. There were no exclusion criteria.

Procedure

Following approval of the Institutional Review Board, data collection began in February 2010. Medical records from all 325 patients who received a TKA during FY 2009 were reviewed by the staff research nurse at the rate of 10 to 20 per month. A study instrument listing 27 risk factors was developed by the core team and used to record all pertinent data from each patient's medical record (see **Table 1**).

As new evidence emerged about risk factors for SSIs, several Institutional Review Board protocol revisions were submitted to include new variables such as preoperative and postoperative glycemic status, presence of urinary catheters, and incidence of urinary tract infection within 48 hours. Medical records that had been reviewed were then rereviewed to be sure that all medical records had been reviewed for the same variables.

Analysis

Once data collection was completed, analysis was conducted using Pearson product moment correlation coefficient and χ^2 with SPSS version 16. Simple frequencies such as gender, age, and ethnicity were used to describe demographic data. Correlations among relevant variables such as age and SSI were explored, as were other interactions such as comorbidities.

RESULTS

Medical records for all cases of TKA during the study period were analyzed. For FY 2009, 10 out of 325, or 3.25% of patients undergoing TKA, were identified with SSIs for risk categories 0 and 1. The mean age of the sample was 67 years, with a range

Table 3 Sample demographics (N = 325)							
Age (y)		**Gender (%)**		**Ethnicity (%)**		**Comorbidities (%)**	
Mean	67	Female	63	Asian	46	Diabetes	24
Range	19-89 years old	Male	37	White	28	Obesity	8
				Native Hawaiian/ Pacific Islander	21	Immunosuppression	6
				Other	5	Previous infection	6

of 19 to 89 years. Most (63%) of the sample was female. Asian-Americans comprised the largest ethnic group (46%), followed by white people (28%) and Native Hawaiians and Pacific Islanders (21%). The predominant comorbidity was diabetes (24%) (**Table 3**).

Although no risk factors were significantly correlated with SSI development, data analysis identified practice variation and nonadherence to the TKA practice standards in the perioperative and postoperative settings. For example, inconsistencies in practice were noted during chart review for dressing changes, skin site preparations, removal of urinary catheters, discontinuation of antibiotics at 24 hours, and hyperglycemia monitoring (**Table 4**).

DISCUSSION

During this descriptive study, new evidence became available regarding the importance of the role of glucose control in the development of SSI in patients receiving TKA. This new evidence coincided with the growing awareness of lack of standardized practices and inconsistent documentation of pertinent data. In particular, no standards existed for the frequency of measuring glucose and, despite the high rate of persons with a comorbidity of diabetes, documentation of glucose was inconsistent in the medical record. Although these inconsistencies became limitations of the study because of the inability to examine glycemia as an independent variable effecting SSI, they also served as a trigger for an EBP project on the same unit.

This study contributed to increased awareness of risk factors associated with SSIs across disciplines. For example, an unexpected consequence of this study was the immediate change in practice implemented by orthopedic surgeons. As the research team began to describe practice related to surgical preparations, many surgeons switched their selection from iodine-based preparations to chlorhexidine gluconate–based surgical preparations, which were more definitely supported by the literature.

The resulting improved registered nurse compliance with implementation of a perioperative bundle (**Table 5**) has led to 10 out of 11 consecutive quarters with zero SSIs for risk categories 0 and 1 in patients receiving a TKA (see **Fig. 2**). Improved standardization of preoperative and postoperative practice standards, establishment of new

Table 4 Documentation compliance	
Documentation in Electronic Medical Record	**Compliance (%)**
Postoperative day of dressing change	98
Urinary catheter removal	89
Glucose check	32

Table 5
Elements of perioperative bundle for SSI Prevention with TKA

Preoperative Phase	Intraoperative Phase	Postoperative Phase	Discharge/Continuing Care Phase
Preoperative class • Early patient participation • Infection prevention • Smoking cessation • Hyperglycemia management • Identification of special needs • MRSA screening	SCIP[a] and other measures • Prophylaxis antibiotics • Skin preparation • Space suits • OR environment • Suture and drain management • Hyperglycemia management	SCIP[a] and other measures • Dressing change at 48 h • Discontinue prophylaxis antibiotic within 24 h • Discontinue urinary catheter on postoperative day 1 • Hyperglycemia management • Out of bed, postoperative day 1 (OT/PT) • Pain management • VTE prophylaxis within 24 h of surgery	Follow-up care • Meet with physicians • Hyperglycemia management • Infection prevention • Prophylaxis dental medication • Follow-up discharge call

Abbreviations: MRSA, methicillin-resistant *Staphylococcus aureus*; OT, occupational therapy; PT, physical therapy; SCIP, Surgical Care Improvement Project; VTE, venous thromboembolism.

[a] Surgical Care Improvement Project (Source: The Joint Commission, Surgical Care Improvement Project, July 2006. http://www.jointcommission.org/surgical_care_improvement_project/).

practice protocols to eliminate SSIs, and fewer variations in practice at the bedside contributed to the results of this study. It also generated the subsequent EBP project that manages glycemia in this population.[9] These collaborative efforts resulted in certification by The Joint Commission Knee Arthroplasty Programs in June 2012.

Several factors contributed to the success of this project. Monthly meetings of the interprofessional team meant that stakeholders were engaged from the outset. In addition, keeping physician colleagues involved in the project planning and team meetings, and updated via surgical executive meetings, led to immediate and steadfast buy-in and fewer barriers when findings highlighted practice variation. Focusing on patient safety kept all team members open to considering risk factors and modifying practice in their respective areas.

Two added benefits resulted from this research project: (1) professional growth of the interprofessional team, and (2) the identification of a gap in the delivery of care for patients receiving joint replacements. The lack of standardization on timing and documentation of glucose values triggered an EBP change that improved the identification and management of hyperglycemia. The process and results of the subsequent EBP project are described in Part II of this series.[9]

SUMMARY

A descriptive study of risk factors for SSI in patients receiving TKA discovered an infection rate higher than the benchmark. Although no risk factors were significant predictors of SSI in this population, an important finding was that, despite a patient population with comorbid diabetes, a lack of standardized practice related to the identification and management of hyperglycemia was identified. These research findings identified and validated an important practice issue and led to the continued commitment to improve glucose management. In this way, a descriptive research study served as a trigger for improved nursing practice using an EBP approach.

REFERENCES

1. Cram P, Lu X, Kates SL, et al. Total knee arthroplasty volume, utilization, and outcomes among Medicare beneficiaries, 1991-2010. JAMA 2012;308:1227–36.
2. Data from the National Hospital Discharge Survey. 2010. Available at: http://www.cdc.gov/nchs/data/nhds/4procedures/2010pro_numberpercentage.pdf. Accessed March 14, 2013.
3. Poultsides LA, Ma Y, Della Valle AG, et al. In-hospital surgical site infections after primary hip and knee arthroplasty - incidence and risk factors. J Arthroplasty 2013;28:385–9.
4. Agos F, Shoda C, Bransford D. Part II: managing peri-operative hyperglycemia in total hip and knee replacement surgeries. 2014.
5. Hanazaki K, Maeda H, Okabayashi T. Relationship between perioperative glycemic control and postoperative infections. World J Gastroenterol 2009;15:4122–5.
6. American Nurses Credentialing Center. Application manual: magnet recognition program. Silver Spring (MD): American Nurses Credentialing Center; 2008.
7. National Healthcare Safety Network of the Centers for Disease Control and Prevention. 2009. Available at: http://www.cdc.gov/nhsn/PDFs/pscManual/9pscSSI current.pdf. Accessed October 1, 2010.
8. Saltzman MD, Nuber GW, Gryzlo SM, et al. Efficacy of surgical preparation solutions in shoulder surgery. J Bone Joint Surg Am 2009;91:1949–53.
9. Bibbo C, Patel DV, Gehrmann RM, et al. Chlorhexidine provides superior skin decontamination in foot and ankle surgery: a prospective randomized study. Clin Orthop Relat Res 2005;438:204–8.
10. AORN Position Statement. 2009. Available at: www.aorn.org/PracticeResources/AORNPositionStatements/. Accessed December 15, 2010.

Part II: Managing Perioperative Hyperglycemia in Total Hip and Knee Replacement Surgeries

Florence Agos, BSN, RN[a,b,*], Casey Shoda, BSN, RN[b],
Deborah Bransford, BSN, RN, CDE[c]

KEYWORDS

- Hyperglycemia • Glycemic control • Surgical site infections
- Joint replacement surgery • Perioperative phases

KEY POINTS

- Hyperglycemia is an independent risk factor for surgical site infections, regardless of history of diabetes.
- Literature supports the monitoring and management of hyperglycemia in the perioperative phases regardless of history of diabetes.
- An evidence-based practice guide for the management of perioperative hyperglycemia assists in the reduction of surgical site infections for patients having total joint replacement surgery.

INTRODUCTION

Evidence indicates that perioperative hyperglycemia management is an important factor in reducing the risk of surgical site infections (SSIs) in all patients regardless of existing history of diabetes.[1] Because patients without preexisting diabetes are not usually monitored for perioperative blood glucose (BG) control, they are at an increased risk for hyperglycemia and subsequently SSIs. Although reducing SSIs is

Funding: This project was partially funded by the Agency for Healthcare Research & Quality, 5R13HS017892; Hawaii State Center for Nursing; and Queen Emma Nursing Institute, The Queen's Medical Center, Honolulu, HI.
Conflict of Interest: None.
[a] Orthopedic Surgery Unit, The Queen's Medical Center, Kamehameha 3 Makai, 1301 Punchbowl Street, Honolulu, HI 96813, USA; [b] Surgical Short Stay Unit, The Queen's Medical Center, Kamehameha 3 Makai, 1301 Punchbowl Street, Honolulu, HI 96813, USA; [c] Patient Care Consulting Services, The Queen's Medical Center, 1301 Punchbowl Street, Honolulu, HI 96813, USA
* Corresponding author. The Queen's Medical Center, Kamehameha 3 Makai, 1301 Punchbowl Street, Honolulu, HI 96813.
E-mail address: fagos@queens.org

Nurs Clin N Am 49 (2014) 299–308
http://dx.doi.org/10.1016/j.cnur.2014.05.004
0029-6465/14/$ – see front matter © 2014 Elsevier Inc. All rights reserved.

nursing.theclinics.com

important for Centers for Medicaid and Medicare Services (CMS) reimbursement, there are additional ramifications that include increased pain, decreased patient satisfaction, increased length of stay, and increased hospital readmissions.[1,2] In addition, patients with hyperglycemia have an 8-fold increase in mortality caused by infectious disorders compared with patients with normoglycermia.[3,4]

To improve perioperative outcomes, hyperglycemic patients must first have their BG monitored, then managed. Hyperglycemia management for this project was defined as maintaining a BG level less than 200 mg/dL.[5,6] The importance of maintaining the recommended BG level within the first 48 hours after surgery is supported in the literature.[7–9]

This article describes the impact of an evidence-based (EB) practice standard for perioperative hyperglycemia management in the reduction of SSIs in patients having total hip and knee replacement surgery. Using the Iowa Model of Evidence-Based Practice to Promote Quality Care, the rationale for this project was to evaluate the impact of EB practices for perioperative hyperglycemia management in the reduction of SSIs in patients having total hip and knee replacement surgery.[10]

Triggers

Reduction of SSIs is one of the quality indicators reported by National Healthcare Safety Networks (NHSN) of the Centers for Disease Control and Prevention (CDC). In 2009 and 2010, the orthopedic surgical unit had an increased number of SSIs, above the CDC benchmark. The preimplementation data showed that there was an increased infection rate among the total joint surgical patients on the orthopedic unit at the facility. For classifying SSIs, the Basic SSI Risk Index was used. This index is issued by the NHSN to assign surgical patients into categories based on the presence of 3 risk factors: (1) operation of longer than average duration; (2) contaminated or dirty/infected wound classification; (3) American Society of Anesthesiologists (ASA) classification of higher risk. The number of total risk factors is the SSI risk category of the patient is shown in **Box 1**.[11] The 2009 SSIs rates for the facility were above the CDC benchmark for patients having both hip and knee replacement. Although there was some improvement in the rates for 2010, they remained above the benchmark (**Figs. 1** and **2**).

Form a Team

The project took place in an acute tertiary health care facility accredited by The Joint Commission (TJC). The facility is licensed for 505 acute beds and 28 subacute beds.

Box 1
Basic SSI risk index

The index used in the NHSN assigns surgical patients into categories based on the presence of 3 major risk factors:

1. Operation lasting more than the duration cut-point hours, where the duration cut point is the approximate 75th percentile of the duration of surgery in minutes for the operative procedure.

2. Contaminated (class 3) or dirty/infected (class 4) wound class.

3. ASA classification of 3, 4, or 5.

The patient's SSI risk category is the number of these factors present at the time of the operation.

Data from Centers for Disease Control and Prevention. Surgical site infection event 2012:14. Available at: http://www.cdc.gov/hai/pdfs/NHSN/9pscSSI-SAMPLE.pdf. Accessed November 12, 2013.

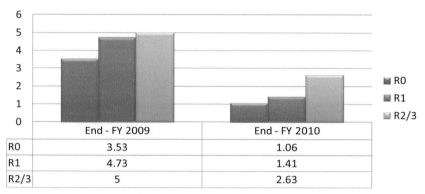

Fig. 1. Medical center's SSI rates for total hip replacement surgeries for risk categories 0, 1, and 2/3. CDC benchmark 2009: R0, 0.28; R1, 1.35; R2, 2.21. CDC benchmark 2010: R0, 0; R1, 0.90; R2, 1.87. FY, financial year.

The hospital is the only one in the state to have achieved Magnet status (the highest institutional honor for hospital excellence) from the American Nurses Credentialing Center. The unit on which the project was piloted and implemented is a 24-bed orthopedic surgical unit that has been awarded the TJC disease certification for hip and knee replacement programs.

A multidisciplinary team developed an EB practice standard for this project. The team comprised 3 orthopedic staff nurses, the orthopedic nurse manager, diabetes nurse educator, diabetes pharmacist, diabetes advance practice nurse, dietitian, hospitalist, endocrinologist, and performance improvement coordinator. The core team consisted of 2 staff nurses, a nurse manager, the performance improvement coordinator, and a diabetes nurse educator. The primary expected outcome was to standardize, using the best available evidence, the practice of hyperglycemia monitoring and management in the preoperative, recovery, and postoperative phases for patients undergoing total knee or hip replacement surgery. Additional anticipated outcomes included standardization of hand-off reports to the patient's primary care physician

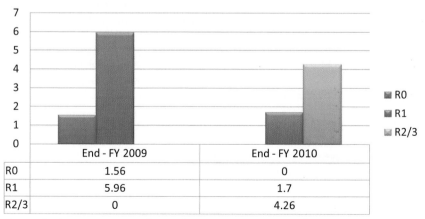

Fig. 2. Medical center's SSI rates for total knee replacement surgeries for risk categories 0, 1, and 2/3. CDC benchmark 2009: R0, 0.32; R1, 0.77; R2, 1.63. CDC benchmark 2010: R0, 0; R1, 0.48; R2, 0.81.

(PCP) after discharge, reduction of SSI rates on the total joint replacement unit, and advancing nurses' knowledge and skills regarding hyperglycemia management of this population.

EVIDENCE FOR PRACTICE IMPROVEMENT
Assemble Relevant Literature

A literature search using PubMed and CINAHL (Cumulative Index to Nursing and Allied Health Literature) databases was completed to identify the evidence for this project. Criteria for including articles in the synthesis were (1) male and female adults greater than or equal to 18 years old; (2) hyperglycemia complications, prevention, and control; (3) SSI after surgery; (4) BG management before and after surgery; (5) complications of strict glycemic control; and (6) follow-up care after surgery. National guidelines published by CDC,[11] the Surgical Care Improvement Project,[12] and the American Diabetes Association[13] were also searched for additional references.

Critique and Synthesize Research

Thirty-eight articles from 2000 to 2013 were critiqued using Mosby levels of evidence and synthesized (**Table 1**). The search terms used were glycemic control, hyperglycemia, perioperative phases, BG, hemoglobin A1c, postoperative SSI(s), joint replacement surgeries, and diabetes mellitus (DM). The relationship between hyperglycemia and SSIs was prevalent throughout the literature. The literature reported that patients with and without a diagnosis of DM are at risk for hyperglycemia, particularly in the first 48 hours after surgery.[1,7] Furthermore, persistent hyperglycemia in the hospitalized patient should be managed like DM.[14,15] The evidence supported a premeal BG level less than 100 mg/dL and a postprandial level less than 180 mg/dL as an ideal target.[14] However, avoidance of hypoglycemia when using insulin to manage hyperglycemia was emphasized repeatedly, especially while the patient is not yet consuming food or drink.[1,2,16]

Other findings suggested that an insulin sliding-scale regimen alone is not an effective therapy for improving BG, and that hemoglobin A1c is not an important indicator in the reduction of SSIs.[5,17] In addition, the Department of Health and Human Services considers manifestations of poor glycemic control as a hospital-acquired condition. Patients who experience prolonged hyperglycemia during hospitalization require discharge follow-up with their PCP because further assessment is needed to differentiate between a diagnosis of stress hyperglycemia and diabetes.[13]

Table 1
Mosby levels of evidence

Mosby Level	Description	Number of Articles
Level I	Meta-analysis	1
Level II	Experimental design (randomized control trial)	4
Level III	Quasiexperimental design	1
Level IV	Case-controlled, cohort studies; longitudinal studies	13
Level V	Correlation studies	6
Level VI	Descriptive studies	1
Level VII	Authority opinion or expert committee reports	2
Other	Performance improvements; review of literature	10

Adapted from Melnyk B. A focus on adult acute and critical care. Worldviews Evid Based Nurs 2004;1(3):194–7; with permission.

IMPLEMENTATION STRATEGIES

Evidence supported monitoring and managing BG in all 3 phases of the perioperative setting. Chart reviews indicated that most patients with prior history of diabetes had orders for monitoring blood sugars once on the orthopedic surgical unit, but not always in the preoperative holding and immediate postoperative areas. In addition, patients without a diagnosis of diabetes had no orders to monitor BG in these areas.

Pilot the Change in Practice

The core team determined that the evidence was sufficient to guide a practice change and created an EB practice standard/guide. The basic element of the guide was a new order set incorporated in the electronic medical record (EMR) to include monitoring and management of hyperglycemia of diabetic and nondiabetic patients having total knee and hip replacement. This order set assisted the physician in selecting orders based on the patients' known or unknown history of diabetes. The practice standard was reviewed and accepted by the hospital's nursing and medical governing committees. To simplify the EB guide, an algorithm was created and used as the primary means of educating the nursing staff (**Fig. 3**).

An implementation strategy was developed to pilot the practice change on the affected units: anesthesia preoperative evaluation center (APEC), preoperative unit, postanesthesia care unit (PACU), and the orthopedic surgery unit. An assessment of the nurses' knowledge regarding effects of hyperglycemia in surgical patients was conducted through a brief questionnaire before the education portion of the pilot. Education sessions, including in-services, emails, and flyers, were provided to all stakeholders (users of the EB standard). These stakeholders included nurses and nurse managers on the units listed earlier, as well as nursing assistants (NAs), dietitians, pharmacists, the orthopedic surgeons and their residents, anesthesiologists, and hospitalists. One endocrinologist was an ad hoc team member and the 2 other endocrinologists who covered the medical center were informed via a letter that included a copy of the EB guide. In addition, the patients were educated about the new practice change by modification of the existing preoperative teaching class offered to patients having elective total hip and knee replacements.

Because the most dynamic change to practice was obtaining a point of care (POC) BG test on all patients having hip and knee replacement surgery, it was decided that creating order sets in the EMR would best facilitate compliance with this practice change. Monitoring of the BG started on arrival at the preoperative holding area and continued through postoperative day (POD) 3. In the preoperative holding area and the PACU, the blood sugar was checked once. For patients without history of diabetes, the checks were done twice daily on PODs 0 to 3. For patients with diabetes, the checks were 4 times daily on PODs 0 to 3. All patients were checked, regardless of whether or not they had a diagnosis of diabetes. If a patient experienced 2 occurrences of a BG level greater than 200 mg/dL, the surgeon was notified. The surgeon would then make a decision to consult the hospitalist and/or the inpatient diabetes team who would assume management of the patient's BG.

In addition to the POC testing, the order sets included notification of the anesthesia provider. Existing postoperative order sets for physicians were modified to incorporate an order to monitor patients without prior history of DM. A discharge template was created to assist nursing staff in communicating with the patient's PCP that follow-up was recommended to assess persistent hyperglycemia (**Box 2**).

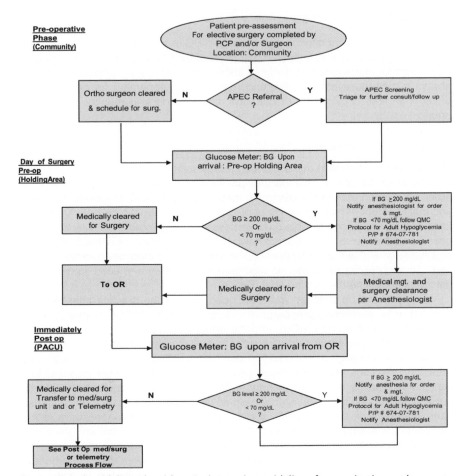

Fig. 3. Clinical guideline algorithm. Perioperative guidelines for monitoring and management of hyperglycemia for joint replacement (hip and knee) surgery. APEC, anesthesia pre-operative evaluation center; N, no; OR, operating room; P/P, policies/procedures; QMC, the queen's medical center; Y, yes.

The practice change was piloted for 3 months. Nurses and physicians were encouraged to provide written feedback on any concerns or problems during the pilot phase. The staff members were also encouraged to discuss concerns with the team members assigned to their unit. The team devised resolutions to the expressed concerns and communicated modifications to the stakeholders. The EB standard/guide was revised accordingly before full implementation, as described later.

Box 2
Discharge note template

This patient was admitted to [unit] from *** to ***. During this admission the patient's blood glucose was increased to more than 200 mg/dL. Because of hyperglycemia episodes the patient was treated with ***. The patient was instructed to present to the PCP for follow-up within 7 days of discharge.

*** Denotes free text area to be completed by the nurse.

EVALUATION
Staff

A major concern that arose during the pilot phase was the increased workload on nursing staff in performing POC BG testing on the patients having total hip and knee replacement. NAs on the orthopedic unit were offered POC glucose meter training. This training was voluntary, because it is currently not a job requirement for that position. The nurse manager authorized a new shift start time for the NAs to assist in performing fasting BG tests on these patients. This new time was found not only to lighten the nurses' workload but to have the added effect of increasing the NAs' involvement with the practice change.

Noncompliance with using order sets was another anticipated issue. The orthopedic surgeons' and residents' compliance improved after several reminders to the surgeons and their residents. The posteducation questionnaire of nurses' knowledge indicated improved understanding of the effects of hyperglycemia in this patient population. Adherence to the guideline for BG screening was 89% during the preoperative phase and 96% in the immediate postoperative recovery phase. The result of this practice change identified 10 patients (7%) as having persistent hyperglycemia and these patients were monitored and managed throughout their inpatient stays. During the pilot phase there were no related hypoglycemic episodes in these patients. The standardization of hand-off reports to the PCP was accomplished for 7 of the 10 patients identified as having persistent hyperglycemia.

Impact of Practice Change

As suggested in the literature, the postpilot data indicated that the guideline may have contributed to reducing the risk for SSIs and improving the safety of this patient population. The facility's comparative data on patients having total hip and knee replacement collected for SSIs from fiscal year (FY) 2009 to the second quarter of FY 2012 reflects a reduction in SSI rate for all risk categories (SSI rate per 100 cases using CDC/NHSN criteria) (**Figs. 4** and **5**).

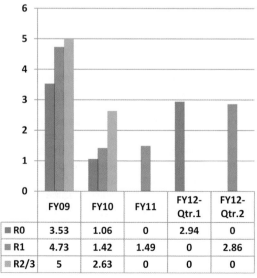

	FY09	FY10	FY11	FY12-Qtr.1	FY12-Qtr.2
R0	3.53	1.06	0	2.94	0
R1	4.73	1.42	1.49	0	2.86
R2/3	5	2.63	0	0	0

Fig. 4. Medical center's SSI rates for total hip replacement. Risk categories 0, 1, and 2/3 (see **Box 1**). Comparative data before and after implementation.

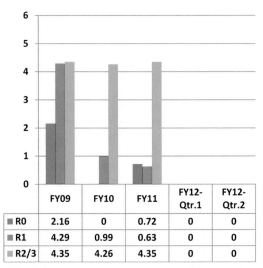

	FY09	FY10	FY11	FY12-Qtr.1	FY12-Qtr.2
▪ R0	2.16	0	0.72	0	0
▪ R1	4.29	0.99	0.63	0	0
▪ R2/3	4.35	4.26	4.35	0	0

Fig. 5. Medical center's SSI rates for total knee replacement. Risk categories 0, 1, and 2/3 (see **Box 1**). Comparative data before and after implementation.

LESSONS LEARNED/RECOMMENDATIONS

Collaboration among the multidisciplinary team and active participation of the staff nurses contributed to the success of this project. Frequent communication with nurse managers, physicians, and the various governing committees was helpful in receiving approval and support for implementation. Monthly meetings with the core team to discuss implementation strategies and revisions of the EB standard were instrumental in keeping stakeholders engaged and moving forward. Ad hoc members were invited to the monthly meetings as necessary to provide feedback on the EB standard and recommendations for the 3-month pilot. One crucial factor for success was having the endocrinologist and chief orthopedic surgeon as ad hoc team members who were able to facilitate support from their physician colleagues.

Education for all stakeholders positively affected the standardization of care in the patients having total hip and knee surgery. In-services were conducted for the APEC, preoperative unit, PACU, orthopedic residents, nursing staff, physicians' assistants, and physicians. These in-services educated each discipline about the EB standard and order sets created in the EMR.

Incorporating order sets and documentation templates into the EMR was invaluable in sustaining this change in practice, as shown by the continued assessment of clinician compliance and decreased SSI rates through intermittent chart audits. These reviews indicate successful and sustained implementation of the practice change.

Barriers to implementation were identified during the pilot phase. These barriers included staff transitioning to the change in daily practice and communicating to the PCP when hyperglycemia occurred on 2 or more occasions. Continued education of the staff eventually led to compliance with the EB standard.

To prevent inconsistencies in practice, the patients having total hip and knee treatment were assigned only to permanent staff who had received training on this practice change. For long-term sustainability, education on this practice change was added to the orientation of all newly hired nurses. Failure to provide the same type of ongoing education to the new residents and surgeons assigned to the unit was a limitation of this project.

Dissemination

The impact of this project also provided opportunities for the EB practice team to present both poster and podium presentations in 2011 and 2012 at the international Pacific Institute of Nursing conference. The project was also presented at a local EB practice workshop and at a state-wide conference.

SUMMARY

There are multiple risk factors for orthopedic SSI. Evidence indicates that modification of these risk factors leads to a decrease in the SSI rate. Studies have shown that hyperglycemia is an independent risk factor for SSI, which is modifiable regardless of a history of diabetes.

The implementation of an EB practice standard for the management of perioperative hyperglycemia in patients having elective hip and knee replacement, regardless of history of diabetes, led to a reduction of SSI over 3 FY in the medical center. In addition, there was improvement in the outcomes of patients without a history of diabetes who experienced hyperglycemia (glucose of $\geq$200 mg/dL) by identifying them as at risk for diabetes and providing them with continuity of care after their hospital stay.

This EB practice project increased awareness of the importance of hyperglycemia monitoring and management. Staff nurses and NAs developed a greater understanding of their roles in influencing care and patient outcomes from the bedside. The multidisciplinary team modified the practice and the sustainability of the changes has reduced the risk for SSIs and improved the quality and safety for these patients having orthopedic surgery.

ACKNOWLEDGMENTS

The authors acknowledge Michele Hadano, MS, RN, CCRN; Edna Dasalla, RN, BSN, MBA, CRRN; and Mary Sadler, PharmD, CDE for their support of this project.

REFERENCES

1. Hanazaki K, Maeda H, Okabayashi T. Relationship between perioperative glycemic control and postoperative infections. World J Gastroenterol 2009;15(33): 4122–5.
2. Grey N, Perdrizet G. Reduction of nosocomial infections in the surgical intensive care unit by strict glycemic control. Endocr Pract 2004;10(2):46–52.
3. Umpierrez G, Isaaca S, Bazargan N, et al. Hyperglycemia: an independent marker of in-hospital mortality of patients with undiagnosed diabetes. J Clin Endocrinol Metab 2002;87(3):978–82.
4. Campbell K. Etiology and effect on outcomes of hyperglycemia in hospitalized patients. Am J Health Syst Pharm 2007;64(6):S4–8.
5. Marchant M, Viens N, Cook C, et al. The impact of glycemic control and diabetes mellitus on perioperative outcomes after total joint arthroplasty. J Bone Joint Surg Am 2009;91:1621–9.
6. Lamloun S, Mobasher L, Karar A, et al. Relationship between postoperative infectious complications and glycemic control for diabetic patients in an orthopedic hospital in Kuwait. Med Princ Pract 2009;18:447–52.
7. Aragon D, Ring C, Covelli M. The influence of diabetes on postoperative infections. Crit Care Nurs Clin North Am 2003;15(1):125–35.
8. Anderson D, Kaye K, Classen D, et al. Strategies to prevent surgical site infections in acute care hospitals. Infect Control Hosp Epidemiol 2008;29(1):S51–61.

9. Trussel J, Gerkin R, Coates B, et al. The impact of a patient care pathway protocol on surgical site infection rates in cardiothoracic surgery patients. Am J Surg 2008;196(6):883–9.

10. Titler MG, Kleiber C, Steelman VJ, et al. The Iowa model of evidence-based practice to promote quality care. Crit Care Nurs Clin North Am 2001;13(4):497–509.

11. National Healthcare Safety Network for the Centers of Disease Control and Prevention. 2009. Available at: www.cdc.gov/nhsn/PDFs/pscManual/9pscSSIcurrent.pdf. Accessed May 1, 2010.

12. The Joint Commission Surgical Care Improvement Project. 2012. Available at: http://www.jointcommission.org/surgical_care_improvement_project/. Accessed May 1, 2010.

13. American Diabetes Association. Standards of medical care in diabetes 2011. Diabetes Care 2011;34(1):S11–61.

14. Boucher J, Swift C, Franz M, et al. Inpatient management of diabetes and hyperglycemia: implications for nutrition practice and the food and nutrition professional. J Am Diet Assoc 2007;107(1):105–11.

15. Rizvi A, Chillag S, Chillag K. Perioperative management of diabetes and hyperglycemia in patients undergoing orthopaedic surgery. J Am Acad Orthop Surg 2010;18(7):426–35.

16. Smith D, Bowen J, Bucher L, et al. A study of perioperative hyperglycemia in patients with diabetes having colon, spine, and joint surgery. J Perianesth Nurs 2009;24(6):362–9.

17. Moghissi E. Addressing hyperglycemia from hospital admission to discharge. Curr Med Res Opin 2010;26(3):589–98.

Decreasing Inpatient Length of Stay at a Military Medical Treatment Facility

Allison Ferro, RN-BC*, Katrina Mullens, RN-BC, Seth Randall, RN

KEYWORDS

- Inpatient • Length of stay • Evidence-based practice • Discharge planning

KEY POINTS

- Discharge planning is defined as the development of an individualized plan early in the hospital stay for the patient and family before leaving the hospital.
- National and organizational priorities and trends indicated a need to reduce the length of stay in this large urban military medical center.
- Many hospital readmissions are unnecessary or preventable through coordinated, early discharge planning.

INTRODUCTION

Discharge planning is defined as the development of an individualized plan early in the hospital stay for the patient and family before leaving the hospital. The aim of discharge planning is to reduce length of stay and readmission to the hospital, and improve the coordination of services following discharge from the hospital. Of the 39.5 million hospital discharges per year, 19% of patients have a postdischarge adverse event, and 20% of Medicare patients are readmitted within 30 days according to The Centers for Medicaid and Medicare Services.[1] Many hospital readmissions are unnecessary or preventable through coordinated, early discharge planning.

The Joint Commission policy[2] states that discharge planning must occur by planning for services to meet client needs, but does not designate the frequency with which it is to occur (Standard LD.03.03.01, LD.04.03.01, LD.04.04.03, PC.4.100, PC.5.60, PC.6.140, PC.6.170). Improving the effectiveness of communication among caregivers is a National Patient Safety Goal (NPSG) for 2012, which could lead to improved efficiency of discharge. Reducing the risk of health care–associated infections is another NPSG that can be targeted by timely discharge. Some of the

The views expressed in this publication are those of the author(s) and do not reflect the official policy or position of the Department of the Army, Department of Defense, or the US Government.

Disclosure: Commercial support was received in part from the Hawaii State Center for Nursing.

Medical Oncology, Tripler Army Medical Center, 1 Jarrett White Road, Honolulu, HI 96859, USA

* Corresponding author.

E-mail address: allison.l.ferro.mil@mail.mil

organizational priorities with the potential to be positively affected by changes in discharge planning include: (1) improved quality, outcome-focused care, and services; (2) implementation of best practices; (3) improved internal and external communication; and (4) optimized resources and value.[3]

The nursing staff on the inpatient medicine wards of a large urban military medical center noticed the extended length of stay for patients for various reasons, mainly social or financial. Staff nurses were concerned about potential complications and inefficiencies associated with a prolonged hospital stay. These concerns were brought to Unit Practice Council to see whether a more efficient process could be developed for discharge planning.

During fiscal year 2012, this center experienced a loss in revenue based on the Performance-Based Adjustment Model (PBAM)[4] because patients stayed longer than the length of stay expected for their diagnoses. PBAM is designed to modify the resources of military medical centers based on actual medical practices and outcomes rather than performance goals. In addition to the lost revenue, the medical center would incur the cost of an inpatient bed day, which is approximately $3000 per day for an average inpatient stay on a medical-surgical ward.[4] Furthermore, there are risks associated with extended hospitalization, including the risk of hospital-acquired conditions such as pressure ulcers or infections, which can significantly add to the cost of a hospital stay.

National and organizational priorities and trends indicated a need to reduce the length of stay in this large hospital. This article describes an evidence-based practice approach to decreasing the length of stay of inpatient adults on a medicine oncology floor in this medical center.

With the background and triggers identified, an evidence-based practice (EBP) team was formed, which included the team leader, the Clinical Nurse Officer in charge of the medicine oncology ward, the EBP mentor, a Clinical Nurse Specialist, a clinical staff nurse, and 2 physician champions. The EBP team attended the Hawaii State Center for Nursing Internship to acquire a baseline understanding of EBP and to help develop the problem statement. The Iowa Model for Evidence-Based Practice, introduced at the internship, guided the team through the process.[5] A problem statement was developed: "What is the best evidence-based method to plan for discharge early in the hospital stay to improve patient outcomes and decrease length of stay?" The target population was inpatient adults in the Department of Medicine, Medicine Oncology ward. The outcomes of interest were decreased risk of complications during hospitalization, decreased length of stay, and cost savings, in comparison with the previous informal method of discharge planning.

EVIDENCE FOR PRACTICE IMPROVEMENT

A literature search was conducted to assemble and critique relevant research related to discharge planning. Searching the databases of CINAHL and PubMed using the keywords "length of stay," "discharge planning," "patient discharge," and "inpatient adults," the team found 59 articles within the past 10 years that were relevant to the project. Twenty-eight articles were chosen and reviewed using the nursing research evidence appraisal tool developed by Johns Hopkins to grade the varying levels of evidence (**Table 1**). The articles reviewed were of varying evidence levels, the highest being Level I, which is a randomized controlled trial or a meta-analysis of a randomized controlled trial. Level II signifies a quasi-experimental study, and Level III is a nonexperimental or qualitative study.

There was strong evidence to suggest that formalized discharge planning rounds would benefit the target patient population.[6] In addition, the use of a discharge

Table 1	
Johns Hopkins nursing research evidence appraisal tool	
Level of Evidence	**Number of Articles Found**
I	5
II	8
III	15
Average level of evidence: 2.35	Total articles: 28

advocate (DA) was shown to be successful at the Mayo Clinic.[7] Having strong physician champions as supporters of the discharge-planning rounds led to strong buy-in from the interdisciplinary care team, and overall support for the change.

Staff Perspective

To the staff, there was a perceived need to formalize discharge planning because they noticed that many patients were staying for months at a time. The staff was acutely aware of the risk to those patients who were hospitalized past the acute stage of their illness. The patients who were staying past their recommended length of stay often had a high nursing acuity level of care, with comorbidities of dementia or other end-of-life concerns that are often difficult to manage at home. Some of the patients died before they could be discharged. The staff wanted to provide the best possible care for these patients, which was leading to an increased staffing burden and a parallel increased risk for burnout because staff members were not witnessing progress toward discharge. The staff was working diligently to prevent complications rather than to return the patient to a state of wellness.

The staff also became attached to patients who were hospitalized in one location for a long period as they became part of the unit. The staff members felt responsible for creating a discharge plan or helping to achieve discharge; however, they did not know what their resources were and did not feel equipped to handle this complex patient population. It was time-consuming to tackle a complicated discharge and, owing to shift work, the efforts were often disjointed. The Clinical Nurse Officer in charge was highly involved with each long-stay patient, and became a proponent for change, which led to increased communication among the staff. In addition, a need for a proper location in which to document the discharge plan was identified. A note was created in the electronic medical record to document the barriers to discharge, and the planning that was occurring.

Administrative Priorities

From an administrative perspective, the backlog of patients at the lowest acuity level of care on the medical-surgical ward was creating a problem for the monitored beds and intensive care units. Pressure was put on the management of the medical-surgical wards to open up bed space so that other areas of the medical center in high demand did not have to go on divert. The backlog that was stopping patient flow from high levels of care needed to be addressed, starting at the lowest level. Because of the frequent need to divert the higher-acuity patients, the entire chain of command was attempting to find a solution to this complex issue.

Through the efforts of the interdisciplinary team, there was an increase in awareness of the importance of improved discharge planning. The length of stay was being closely tracked by number of days, and was clearly displayed on the ward to bring awareness to the staff. This point marked the start of the cultural change on the ward regarding discharge planning. Staff nurses were encouraged to advocate for the patient by pursuing updates on discharge on a daily basis. The charge nurse incorporated the discharge needs into the daily shift change that was updated twice a day. Greater pressure was placed on the interdisciplinary team to provide updates for each patient's plan of care. The culture was slowly changing from being complacent about the lack of timely discharge to being strong patient advocates using formalized discharge planning. This culture change took place early on in the process and was supported by the entire interdisciplinary team, which led to success of the initiative. Success was further enhanced by early dissemination of project findings in addition to having 2 physician champions on the team to encourage physician acceptance of the project and related changes in practice.

IMPLEMENTATION STRATEGIES
Discharge-Planning Meeting

Because the team thought it important to have input from all disciplines to achieve success, discharge-planning meetings were started in April 2012. Every member of the interdisciplinary team was included: social work, case management, physical therapy, chaplain, clinical nurse specialist, utilization management, charge nurse or clinical nurse officer in charge, and physician team members.

The meeting was scheduled weekly on the inpatient medicine oncology ward to bring together the interdisciplinary team to discuss barriers to discharge for patients initially who had a length of stay of 30 days or longer. After 2 months the interdisciplinary team saw the benefits of discussing these patients, and decided to discuss every patient admitted to the ward. The meetings were well organized and well attended. Every attempt was made to keep the meeting short so that attendance would continue and patient care would not be negatively affected. Meetings normally lasted 1 hour, with each of the 4 inpatient physician teams attending in approximately 15-minute increments.

Documentation

At the start of the EBP project, an interdisciplinary discharge-planning note was created in the electronic medical record to document what was discussed at the meeting. The note contained basic information about the patient, current barriers to discharge, expected discharge location, equipment needed, and documentation of the weekly discussion of the patient's discharge plan. The note was initially filled out by the clinical nurse officer in charge to prevent an additional documentation burden on the nursing staff. Any member of the team could read or contribute to the note as necessary. This note became a useful way to keep the team informed of the patient's progress toward discharge. Later the note was used to collect baseline data regarding barriers to discharge that were used to create the evidence-based guideline and pilot program.

Discharge Advocate

As part of the Iowa Model for Evidence-Based Practice,[4] a trial of the desired intervention based on the literature was piloted to ascertain whether the change would affect the desired outcomes (Appendix 1). The intervention chosen was the use of a DA, and an evidence-based guideline was written to specify the scope of responsibility for this role (see Appendix 1). The screening that the DA would conduct was modeled after a project that was previously conducted called project RED or Re-Engineered Discharge, from the Agency for Healthcare Research and Quality.[8]

The DA screened every patient for barriers to discharge on admission. The DA was also responsible for rounding with physician teams daily to clarify the plan of care and then to discuss and modify the plan with the patient, as needed. The DA worked with family members to obtain useful information regarding discharge needs and to educate them regarding the plan. The DA was responsible for initiating and documenting discharge planning and for improving planning meetings for the ward.

The DA became the liaison within the interdisciplinary team to coordinate every discharge. The staff approached the DA to troubleshoot complex discharge issues that required an excessive amount of time or resources. The physician teams felt comfortable communicating with one subject-matter expert for discharge planning instead of attempting to communicate with different staff nurses. The DA was a good resource for the physicians in helping to determine the barriers to discharge from the patient's perspective that had not been communicated.

One example of a barrier to discharge that was identified as a result of the pilot program was a timing issue with laboratory blood draws. Draw samples were not being collected early enough to be assessed in time for the morning physician rounds, thus delaying discharge decisions, sometimes causing the patient to stay an extra day. After implementation of the program, if a patient was identified as a possible discharge for the following day the laboratory blood draws would be collected before 4 AM to enable processing in time for physician rounds. The decision for discharge could then be made early enough to coordinate all the necessary steps for discharge.

Changing the Culture

Several education strategies were used so that the project was visible at all levels. Throughout the project, every opportunity was used to create visibility and gain support at all levels. At an early stage of the project, the Department of Medicine key leadership team was briefed on the creation of the project and its initial progress. Members of the team were educated on the problem and background so that they understood the overall project. During this presentation, the physician champions were identified to show that there was early physician support. The presentation created awareness throughout the department and began the process of obtaining support from the leadership.

After the project was planned and the pilot initiated, the nursing staff was made aware of the project. At a staff meeting, the DA was introduced and the concept discussed, and the role of the DA was explained. Shortly after implementation, positive feedback was received from the nurses. Even the staff members who were resistant at the beginning became advocates for change after seeing the positive aspects of the pilot. Monthly updates during staff meetings were provided to the staff as the project continued.

Every opportunity was used to create awareness for the project throughout the medical center. The team members presented the project during Nursing Grand Rounds in December 2012. These continuing education presentations are facility wide, and are open to all staff. The project was also presented to key leadership at the EBP updates seminar attended by both the Deputy Commander for Nursing and the Chief Nurse. At both presentations, the project generated positive feedback and created even more visibility. A poster was presented at Nurses Week in May 2013 to display visual results of the project, and was later displayed on the ward.

EVALUATION

The outcomes selected for evaluation were inpatient length of stay and estimated savings. Other outcomes initially considered for evaluation were hospital-acquired pressure ulcers and hospital-acquired infections. The rate for hospital-acquired infections in this particular ward was very low, so a comparison before and after implementation would have been insignificant. The origin of hospital-acquired infections is difficult to determine because of multiple interward transfers, so this outcome was not selected for use. Therefore, length of stay and estimated savings were used to measure the effectiveness of this EBP project.

Length of Stay

During the initial 65 days of the pilot, every patient's length of stay was tracked. The length of the pilot was determined by the availability of the first DA. Because of the high turnover in the military population, the initial DA was only available for the initial period of the pilot, but was then replaced. Patients' actual length of stay was compared with their admission diagnosis code. More than 417 days were identified whereby patients were hospitalized past the estimated length of stay. Before the pilot, detailed baseline data were not collected so that a direct comparison could be made once the pilot began. However, the authors were able to assume that length of stay decreased because, during the pilot, admissions increased while the census decreased. The average daily census went from 20 patients to 12 patients in a 30-day span (**Fig. 1**). These findings were consistent with those found in the literature.

When identifying how long patients were staying, the team found that 3% of patients were staying longer than 30 days, 58% of patients were staying between 2 and 30 days, and 34% of patients were staying for less than 1 day, which was an unexpected finding (**Fig. 2**). Even though the DA was focusing on only 3% of patients, these patient stays made up most of the overall bed days and were the principal contributor to the fines that were identified as a problem by the chain of command. When the pilot findings were presented to the chain of command, it was determined that the DA role was necessary, and the leadership supported the long-term implementation of the program. A future area of investigation might be the population who were staying less than 1 day. The project helped identify these groups and bring awareness of them to the chain of command.

Cost Savings

Potential cost savings were identified during this pilot project. An average hospital bed day costs approximately $957.[9] There were 417 excess bed days identified over the course of the pilot, which equates to an estimated $399,069 in potential cost savings

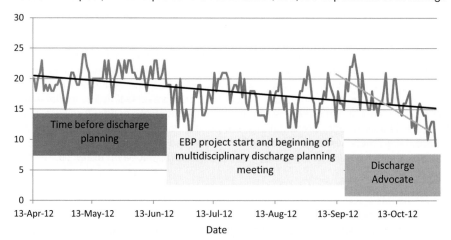

Fig. 1. Medicine Oncology patient census over time. EBP, evidence-based practice.

Days Spent in Hospital N=276

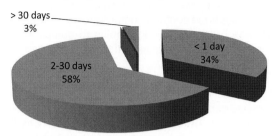

> 30 days
3%

2-30 days
58%

< 1 day
34%

Fig. 2. Medicine Oncology length of stay breakdown.

during the length of the pilot alone. Extrapolated over a year, if the use of a DA was adopted as a full-time position, there is a potential annual cost savings of $2,240,925. This figure does not account for potential cost savings associated with decreasing risk of hospital-acquired complications associated with increased length of stay. For example, it is estimated that a single hospital-acquired pressure ulcer can cost between $20,900 and $151,700.[10] In addition, by decreasing average length of stay there is an increased opportunity for cost savings attributable to the ability to care for more patients, open nonmonitored beds, and prevent the hospital from going on divert.

Discharge Advocate Revisions

Owing to personnel transfers, the original DA was replaced after the initial 65 days. The initial DA role was adapted based on the needs of the pilot, and was adapted later again because of a change in personnel. One change that occurred was that the second DA moved the location of his office to the ward to increase visibility, which also improved communication between the staff and the physicians. The second DA was more involved with the actual discharge of the patients, thereby shifting the workload of discharging patients from the nurses. Another implemented change was that the DA began making follow-up phone calls to the patients before their follow-up appointment. As a result of the work of the DAs and the presentation of results to the leadership, a decision was made to make the DA position permanent on this ward. Other wards in the facility are looking to mimic the use of a DA in specialty populations such as patients undergoing total joint replacement.

Barriers to Discharge

The main barriers to discharge that were identified by pulling data from the interdisciplinary discharge-planning note were transportation, housing, social situations regarding placement, the ability to receive intravenous antibiotics, Medicaid paperwork approval, and patient refusal. All of these barriers are related directly to the culture of the military health care system in which patients are accustomed to minimal out-of-pocket expenses for health care. Depending on the status of the patient (Veteran, Active Duty, Retiree), different levels of benefits are offered. Many times patients did not have money to pay for their own transportation, copays, or housing, which created a delay in discharge. The lack of support systems attributable to geographic isolation or social situations increased the burden on the facility. An inpatient stay for these patients incurred no cost to them, whereas the discharge location would often incur a cost that often created a delay in or refusal to discharge.

As a result of identifying these barriers, the team was able to formulate solutions to some of the common ones. Working groups were formed, which brought these issues up the chain of command for troubleshooting. Many of these issues were solved so that a delay in discharge was not necessary. One example of a solution to a common barrier was the use of a separate contract company to handle the Medicaid paperwork for patients, which was previously taking months to complete. When the contract company took over the Medicaid application, the process became more streamlined.

Impact on Nursing Staff

The nursing staff was satisfied with the outcome of the project because nurses saw tangible progress toward decreasing overall length of stay, especially for those patients with long-term inpatient stays. The staff considered that the DA was a helpful role in troubleshooting difficult discharges, and was acutely aware of and more energized about discharging patients with challenging situations. The nurses now trusted that they had the resources to solve problems instead of feeling burdened by these situations.

LESSONS LEARNED AND RECOMMENDATIONS

The biggest factor that led to the success of the project was the Hawaii State Center for Nursing Internship. The internship's bimonthly meetings were invaluable for holding team members accountable and motivating the team to complete assignments on time. The internship also created a supportive community of nurses from different facilities who shared challenges and solutions related to length of stay and patient discharge. Within individual teams, members from different disciplines created a culture of diversity that led to creative solutions to problems encountered, and enhanced the outcomes of the project. Diversity within the EBP team was also an important part of influencing change within the organization, specifically the experience and influential characteristics of the change champion.

Another key to success was the support received from the leadership. The foundation was developed when the chain of command supported attendance at the Hawaii State Center for Nursing Internship, and continued as they were informed of the project's growth. The project was supported by the chain of command largely because the project measured cost outcomes, an important factor in gaining institutional support.

Challenges

The greatest challenge was the long-term sustainability of the project over time, for a variety of reasons. Staff turnover in a military facility is always high and many team members, staff members, the DA, and leadership changed during the course of the project, slowing down progress despite the team's commitment to moving forward. For future projects it might be helpful to have at least 1 civilian team member to create continuity and serve as an advocate for the project.

Institutional Changes

Lessons were also learned during the stage of the project whereby institutional changes were required. During this phase, support from the chain of command was essential. The command was receptive to the technique of grass-roots change; therefore, the team witnessed greatest success and progress by keeping the chain of command informed at every step of the project. Disseminating the information to stakeholders at all phases of the project was also integral to keeping every level of staff engaged in the success of the project. Despite the Medicine Oncology ward becoming the model for discharge planning, and serving as a resource for discharge planning and documentation throughout the medical center, the discharge process remains difficult to standardize on diverse wards with different patient populations. Evidence may help guide improvements to the discharge process and, at the very least, documentation could be standardized and streamlined to cut down on repetitive charting. For example, other areas of the medical center reevaluated their discharge process and adopted certain aspects of the team's recommendations. However, no other ward adopted the use of a DA, or used the model designed on the Medicine Oncology ward.

Pilot Phase

Military turnover limited the time frame of the pilot phase. The small amount of data that was collected made it difficult to make a concrete comparison before and after implementation of the DA. It was also difficult to compare data by inpatient ward, because most data were available for comparison by diagnosis rather than by ward. Despite limited data collection, the team was able to identify barriers to discharge that could be focused on for future problem solving. The team was able to identify smaller issues and interventions that had a large impact on length of stay, such as the need for transportation services for patients who are unable to use public transportation for medical reasons. Smaller changes were easier to tackle in comparison with larger issues requiring a longer time frame to rectify. Even if the use of a DA is not feasible in a different setting, it is recommended that baseline data be collected on barriers to discharge so that trends can be identified for future process improvement.

Other Recommendations

One recommendation from the literature that was not piloted was the use of a Nurse Practitioner (NP) as the DA.[11] Although the use of an NP was not tested during this pilot project, the benefits discussed in the literature were reportedly beneficial, and would be worthwhile to consider if conducting a similar pilot. The ability of an NP to prescribe discharge medications, interpret diagnostic studies and laboratory tests, and assist with patient teaching could be a beneficial part of the role of a DA.

SUMMARY

The purpose of this article is to describe an evidence-based approach to decreasing the length of stay of inpatient adults on the Medicine Oncology ward of a large urban military medical center. The Iowa Model for Evidence-Based Practice[4] was used to guide the team through the process. A strong and diverse team was formed, which worked together for the duration of the project. The literature recommended formalized discharged planning meetings with a dedicated individual as the planner, coupled with solid documentation.

The significant finding of the project was that the use of a DA in addition to weekly discharge-planning meetings leads to a decrease in the average length of stay on inpatient Medicine Oncology wards. This approach resulted in a cost savings for the facility, derived mainly from a decrease in fines for excessive length of stay. The strongest implication is that a bottom-up approach using strong evidence and a formalized approach can overcome institutional challenges and make a positive impact on patient care. As a result of this project, nurses also came to recognize the role played by EBP in continuously improving patient outcomes.

ACKNOWLEDGMENTS

The authors would like to acknowledge the following for the support of this project: Hawaii Center for Nursing, Katie Rivera, RN, MS, CCNS, CCRN, Julie Jones, MD, Clifton Layman, DO, Angela Zabko, RN, MSN.

REFERENCES

1. Research, statistics, data & systems. The Centers for Medicaid and Medicare Services. Available at: http://www.cms.gov/. Accessed March 19, 2012.
2. The Joint Commission. Accreditation, health care, certification. Available at: http://www.jointcommission.org/. Accessed April 1, 2012.
3. Anonymous. Pacific regional medical command balanced score card. 2012.
4. Anonymous. Performance based adjustment model handbook. 2013.
5. Titler MG, Kleiber C, Steelman V, et al. The Iowa model of evidence-based practice to promote quality care. Crit Care Nurs Clin North Am 2001;13(4):497–509.
6. Balaban RB, Samuel PA, Woolhandler S. Redefining and redesigning hospital discharge to enhance patient care: a randomized controlled study. J Gen Intern Med 2008;23(8):1228–33.
7. Holland DE, Hemann MA. Continuity of care standardizing hospital discharge planning at the Mayo Clinic. Jt Comm J Qual Patient Saf 2011;37(1):29–36.
8. Re-engineered discharge (RED) toolkit. A research group at Boston University Medical Center. 2013. Available at: https://www.bu.edu/fammed/projectred/. Accessed April 1, 2012.
9. American Health Association Annual Surveys. Hospital adjusted expenses per inpatient day by ownership. The Henry J. Kaiser Family Foundation State Health Facts; 2013.
10. Berlowitz D, VanDeusen Lukas C, Parker V, et al. Preventing pressure ulcers in hospitals: a toolkit for improving quality of care. Agency for Healthcare Research and Quality. Available at: www.ahrq.gov. Accessed December 1, 2013.
11. Finn KM, Heffner R, Chang Y, et al. Improving the discharge process by embedding a discharge facilitator in a resident team. J Hosp Med 2011;6(9):494–500.

APPENDIX 1

SUBJECT: Discharge planning evidence-based practice project pilot study evidence-based practice guideline.

PURPOSE: To outline the job description of the Discharge Advocate (DA), as part of the evidence-based practice project pilot study with the goal of a safe, well-planned discharge.

SCOPE: All patients assigned to Inpatient Medicine Wards

GENERAL:

1. Design: The Iowa Model of Evidence-Based Practice to Promote Quality Care

2. Background:

   a. On a literature review of 24 research articles using the key words "discharge planning," "length of stay," and "inpatient adults," the role of the DA has been shown to be beneficial in decreasing the workload for both physicians and nurses, decreasing the length of stay, preventing readmissions, and improving both patient and staff satisfaction.

   b. As part of the Iowa Model for Evidence-Based Practice, a trial of the desired intervention based on the literature will be piloted to see if the change will affect the desired outcomes.

3. Length of pilot project:

   a. The length of the pilot project will be 65 calendar days. At the end of 65 calendar days, an initial review of the data will be performed to determine if the pilot needs to be continued for an extended period of time.

4. Location of the pilot project:

    a. The pilot project will take place on wards 5C2 and 6C2 only.

5. Scope of service:

    a. The DA will perform the following functions for each adult Department of Medicine patient on 5C2 and 6C2 on admission:

        1. Screen patients for barriers to discharge on admission

        2. Conduct early patient teaching on diagnosis, medications, devices, diet and so forth, and document the teaching was conducted. Provide patient teaching materials

        3. Round with physician teams and clarify the plan of care with the patient afterward. Update Lead Registered Nurse note as needed

        4. Engage family members in the discharge process; obtain contact information

        5. Schedule family meetings or teaching sessions as needed

        6. Assist with making follow-up appointments with patients who see an outside primary care manager

        7. Create and document a plan for how the patient will be transported out of the facility on discharge (privately owned vehicle, taxi, bus, ride from family, handi-van, and so forth) and schedule a time if possible

        8. Create and document a plan for how the patient will be transported to follow-up appointments

        9. Document on the "interdisciplinary discharge-planning note" weekly and as needed, ensuring to update the barriers to discharge

        10. Ensure patient has durable medical equipment or oxygen ordered before the day of discharge

        11. Fill out medication worksheet, and confirm that the patient understands through feedback

        12. Check to see if patient has valuables in the treasury, and ensure they are retrieved during business hours

        13. Ensure the patient has a complete discharge summary, discharge orders, and discharge medications the day before discharge if possible, or at least before the prearranged time for discharge transportation

        14. Ensure patient has all belongings on discharge

        15. Give interactive customer evaluation comment card and DA survey to each patient

6. Monitoring for results:

    a. The average length of stay will be examined by provider (Department of Medicine only) and diagnoses before and after the intervention

    b. 30-day readmission rates will be examined before and after the intervention

    c. The average time of discharge will be examined before and after the intervention

    d. The barriers to discharge (from the interdisciplinary discharge-planning note pilot 5C2/6B1) will be examined before and after the intervention

    e. Patient satisfaction with the DA will be examined

7. Potential risks and benefits:

    a. The potential benefits of discharge planning are decreased length of stay, prevention of readmission, patient and staff satisfaction, and decreased provider burden

    b. There have been no identified risks in any of the studies examined in the literature review, and there are no other foreseen risks

On first meeting with the patient:

- Ask permission to enter the patient's room
- Introduce yourself by name and identify your role as the DA
- Determine if the patient feels well enough to participate
- Ask the patient how he/she prefers to be addressed
- Ask about language preference
- Assess for language assistance needs and contact interpreter services as necessary
- Speak slowly
- Use plain, nonmedical language
- Actively listen; do not interrupt
- Do not overload the patient with lots of information at once; do not try to cover more than 3 key points at a time
- Be attuned to body language
- Offer encouragement
- Express empathy
- Build self-confidence
- Inform them the goal of the DA program: A safe and well-planned discharge from the hospital that reduces the risk of returning to the hospital, and prevents a prolonged stay

Gather the following information from the patient:

- Primary care clinician's name and office location
- Patient's understanding of illness or treatment
- Medication reconciliation
- Name and contact information of family, caregivers, or social support systems
- Determine family involvement, and ability to support patient on discharge
- Medication and food allergies
- Advanced directives (initiate with SWS if needed)
- Durable equipment he/she has or should have at home
- Patient's needs, requests, and receptiveness
- Gaps in the discharge plan
- Determine the best day and time for scheduling appointments
- Discuss transportation options
- Determine if there are any concerns about discharge
- Determine if there are any known barriers to discharge

Preventing Extubation Failures in a Pediatric Intensive Care Unit

Susan Bankhead, MSN, DNP[a,b,*], Kolea Chong, BSN, CCRN[a],
Sally Kamai, RN, MBA-HCM[c]

KEYWORDS

- Extubation • Mechanical ventilation • PICU
- Iowa Model for Evidence-based Practice

KEY POINTS

- Caring for critically ill children from birth to 21 years of age in the pediatric intensive care unit (PICU) requires multiple life-supporting interventions.
- Although mechanical ventilation can be a necessary life-supporting intervention, there are associated complications.
- The reduction of failed extubations in the PICU from 2.47 per 1000 ventilator days to 0.80 per 1000 ventilator days is attributed to the increased collaboration among care providers, use of the ERA checklist, and implementation of the ERA checklist into the work flow.

INTRODUCTION

Caring for critically ill children from birth to 21 years of age in the pediatric intensive care unit (PICU) requires multiple life-supporting interventions. One necessary intervention is the use of mechanical ventilation for children experiencing progressive respiratory distress, such as labored respirations, decreased oxygen saturation, or airway obstruction. Mechanical ventilation includes the process of intubation, placing an endotracheal tube (ETT) through the mouth and into the lungs, and continued interventions to assist with breathing. These interventions continue until the child recovers and is able to support their respiratory needs with or without the use of noninvasive respiratory initiatives.

Although mechanical ventilation can be a necessary life-supporting intervention, there are associated complications. Some of these complications include ventilator-associated pneumonia, lung and upper airway injury, and prolonged length of stays

Disclosure: None.
[a] Pediatric Intensive Care Unit, Kapiolani Medical Center for Women & Children, 1319 Puna-hou Street, Honolulu, HI 96826, USA; [b] Eastern Idaho Regional Medical Center, 3100 Channing Way, Idaho Falls, ID 83404, USA; [c] Clinical Improvement, Hawaii Pacific Health, 55 Merchant Street 26th Floor, Honolulu, HI 96813, USA
* Corresponding author. Pediatric Intensive Care Unit, Kapiolani Medical Center for Women & Children, 1319 Punahou Street, Honolulu, HI 96826.
E-mail address: Susan.bankheaddnp@gmail.com

in the PICU. The risk of complications is positively associated with the length of time on mechanical ventilation.[1] To reduce the risk of complications, a multidisciplinary team of registered nurses (RN), respiratory therapists (RT), and physicians closely monitors the child's respiratory status to ensure that mechanical ventilation is not used longer than necessary.

After the child demonstrates recovery in oxygen saturation, improved respiratory rate and effort, and minimal need for mechanical ventilation, they transition to noninvasive respiratory support. The transition to noninvasive respiratory support involves planning and coordinating the removal of the ETT and mechanical ventilation, referred to as extubation. Unfortunately, not all planned extubations are successful and some children may need the ETT replaced and restarted on mechanical ventilation. Failed extubation is defined in the literature as the need to reintubate the patient within 24 to 72 hours after a planned extubation.[2] Restarting a patient on mechanical ventilation soon after extubation can significantly increase a patient's risk for ventilator complications and mortality.[3]

The objective of this project was to reduce the number of failed extubations in the Kapiolani Medical Center for Women & Children PICU, a 14-bed regional pediatric academic center that serves the children and families of Hawaii and the Pacific Basin. Failed extubation was defined for this project as the need to reintubate within 48 hours after a planned extubation. After evaluating extubation failures in the PICU and reviewing the literature for best practices for prevention of extubation, the team determined that the creation of an extubation readiness checklist and protocol to predict extubation readiness would assist in decreasing the failed extubation rate. This article describes extubation failures in the PICU and the development and implementation of an extubation readiness protocol using the Iowa Model for Evidence-based Practice as a guideline. The Iowa Model consists of processes for implementing evidence into practice, such as critiquing and synthesizing the literature, identifying stakeholders, and recognizing triggers.[4] The extubation protocol was developed excluding children with previous lung injury and/or neuromuscular conditions, which contribute to an increase risk and complexity of planned extubations.

EVIDENCE FOR PRACTICE IMPROVEMENT
Critiquing and Synthesizing the Literature

A literature search was conducted using CINAHL and PubMed databases to identify publications related to pediatric extubation readiness and extubation failure. The following search terms were used: extubation readiness, pediatric extubation, extubation guidelines, and extubation failure. Seven articles related to pediatric extubation were retrieved and reviewed by the team. The articles ranged in level of evidence from one at level II, two at level VI, and four at level VII using Mosby's criteria. In addition, the team reviewed two pediatric extubation guidelines from other pediatric institutions. All of the articles supported the development of a standardized extubation tool and protocol to guide a multidisciplinary team's assessment of readiness for extubation and to reduce the incidence of extubation failure.

Failed extubation results in patients being reintubated and restarted on mechanical ventilation. The risks associated with reintubation are similar to those of mechanical ventilation and include an increased risk for ventilator-associated pneumonia, lung injury, increased length of stay, and increased mortality in some studies on adults.[3] The collective task force of the American College of Chest Physicians, Association of Respiratory Care, and American College of Critical Care Medicine reports that reintubation carries an eight-fold increase for nosocomial pneumonia, and a 6- to 12-fold increase in mortality.[5] The risks associated with reintubation, therefore, support the importance of preventing failed extubations.

Extubation failure rates ranging from 2% to 20% have been reported.[6] Failed extubation rates have been reported to be approximately 16.3% in infants and children.[7] When specific parameters are used to plan extubation, failure rates are reported between 8% and 9%.[8] It is estimated that based on clinical assessment alone only 35% of intubated patients ready for extubation are properly identified. Thus, the American College of Chest Physicians, Association of Respiratory Care, and the American College of Critical Care Medicine task force support the development of an extubation tool and protocol.[5] This task force recommends patients receiving mechanical ventilation for respiratory failure should undergo a formal assessment before the extubation process.

Without the use of a protocol, the decision to extubate is subjective and physician-dependent. Initial assessment of the extubation process in the PICU demonstrated that the planning of extubation involved an uncoordinated bedside assessment of the child's respiratory status. Consideration was given to the initial causes of the respiratory distress and current level of improvement. However, the decision to extubate was primarily physician driven with support from the bedside RN and RT. Once the child had progressed to minimal mechanical ventilator settings for respiratory support and the child's respiratory status was stable, the bedside team began to focus on the extubation process. The criteria used to remove ventilator support included the ability of the child to maintain spontaneous respirations, presence of a cough/gag to protect the airway, and review of the plan of care for the next 24 hours to ensure that there are no procedures that would require intubation.

The lack of collaboration and inconsistencies in the implementation of the criteria contributed to the PICU's failed extubations. Although the decision to extubate was derived from assessment of the child's respiratory status and physician experiences with extubation, the PICU staff was concerned about the number of failed extubations in the PICU. **Fig. 1** displays the number of failed extubations from 2009 to 2012 per 1000 ventilator days.

IMPLEMENTATION STRATEGIES
Identifying the Stakeholders and Recognizing Triggers

A multidisciplinary team of stakeholders consisting of RNs, RTs, the nurse manager, and a physician champion surveyed 8 of 35 care team members of the PICU to evaluate their current perceptions related to the extubation process and extent of multidisciplinary collaboration. Staff response showed 66% of the staff was not comfortable with the current planned extubation procedure in PICU. When asked about inclusion or collaboration with the extubation plan, only 33% of the staff indicated they were included in the decision-making process. The development of an extubation tool was supported by 87% of the staff who responded to the survey.

A retrospective chart review was conducted using the electronic medical record identifying PICU patients who were reintubated within 48 hours and therefore met the project definition of failed extubations. Electronic medical records of children with previous lung injury and/or neuromuscular conditions were excluded from the review because of the complexity of their disease processes. The failed extubation rate per 1000 ventilator days was 2.47 in 2009 and 1.62 in 2010 based on internal data collection and comparable with failed extubation rates reported in the literature.[6-8] Currently, benchmark data are not available for planned failed extubations.

Based on the staff survey results and the retrospective chart review of all failed extubations (with the exclusion of children with previous lung injury and/or neuromuscular

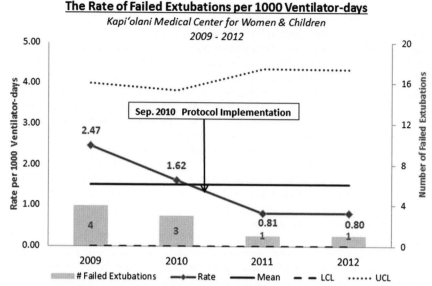

Fig. 1. Rate of failed extubations in the PICU, 2009–2012. LCL, lower control limit; UCL, upper control limit.

conditions), it was determined that a standardized protocol for planned extubation was needed and would be supported by the staff. The standardized approach to planned extubations would address practice inconsistencies and include RN, RT, and physician collaboration with the planned extubations.

The multidisciplinary team created an extubation readiness assessment (ERA) checklist based on published literature and guidelines. This checklist, to be used by the care providers, assists in the determination of readiness for extubation. The newly created ERA checklist includes

- A review of the child's plan of care
- Current ventilator settings
- Level of sedation
- Feeding status
- Presence of a cough/gag
- Child's respiratory effort

Descriptions of predetermined parameters were included on the checklist to assist with and promote standardization in the assessment ERA trial as shown in **Fig. 2**.

Implementing Evidence into Practice

Initiation of the ERA checklist followed a presentation to the PICU intensivists conducted by the physician champion. Because care for the intubated patient includes a multidisciplinary approach, staff education was multifaceted and included team huddles conducted by the managers for the PICU and RT staff. Department-specific education was conducted during staff meetings with the inclusion of the department educators. Individual education was conducted as intubated pediatric patients meeting project criteria were identified during patient rounds as potentially ready for extubation. Individual education was accomplished by assisting the RT and RN in completing the ERA checklist. The ERA checklist was trialed in paper format with

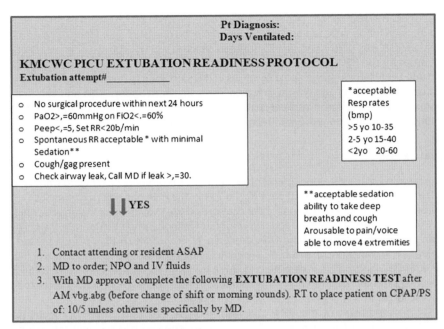

Fig. 2. Sample of the PICU ERA trial tool.

feedback requested and collected from RNs, RTs, and physicians. The feedback, such as best practice alerts and standard physiologic limits, was evaluated by the multidisciplinary team and used to make improvements to the checklist.

At the completion of the ERA checklist trial, a recommendation was made to have the ERA checklist integrated into the electronic medical record. The multidisciplinary team worked with the information technology department to adapt the ERA checklist into the electronic medical record workflow; **Fig. 3** depicts the ERA assessment in the

1100	
Extubation Checklist	
Extubation Attempt #	
Surgical procedure within next 24 hours?	
PaO2 >, = 60mmHg on FiO2 <, = 60%	
Peep <, = 5, Set RR < 20 b/min	
Spontaneous RR acceptable *with minimal	
Cough/gag present	
Call MD if leak >, = 30	
End Tidal CO2 remains < 45 (except CLD pts)	
RR acceptable *with minimal sedation**	
Vt > 5ml/kg (adjust for ideal body weight)	
HR does not increased > 20-40 beats/min	
SaO2 > 92% (unless cyanotic heart lesion)	
SBP > 20 above baseline - resting	
Leak at < 25 cmH2O	
Feeds off for 4 hours	

Fig. 3. PICU extubation readiness checklist converted into the electronic medical record. * reference for acceptable respiratory rates. ** reference for acceptable sedation level.

electronic medical record. The addition of best practice alerts, such as physiologic norms for vital signs based on age, helped make the checklist user friendly. To ensure that an ERA was performed for all intubated children without chronic lung conditions, an order for the ERA was added to the physician intubation order set. This order set included ventilator settings and daily alerts to the care team to perform the ERA checklist when the child progressed to needing less ventilator support. This addition to the order set and electronic medical record created a daily standardized approach for intubated pediatric patients and the plan for extubation (see **Fig. 3**).

EVALUATION

The creation of the ERA checklist tool (see **Fig. 3**) and protocol (see **Fig. 2**) was adopted into practice for children of the PICU in 2011. The ERA checklist systematically incorporates the clinical judgment of the care providers, evaluation of the child's clinical respiratory status, and encourages collaboration among the clinical team in the child's plan of care. A resurvey of the RNs and RTs (N = 6 of 32) in the PICU indicated a decrease in variation of extubation practice among the care provider team from 66% to 0%, and collaboration among the care team increased from 33% to 66%. This outcome demonstrated an improvement in the care team's collaboration and a decrease in the variation of the extubation assessment.

The incorporation of the ERA checklist into the electronic medical record has created a standardized approach for identifying when a child has met the extubation readiness criteria. A review of all PICU failed extubations for children without previous lung injury and/or neuromuscular conditions was conducted at the end of the ERA checklist trial that lasted 14 months. These results demonstrated an overall reduction in failed extubations from 2.47 per 1000 ventilator day in 2009 and 1.67 per 1000 ventilator day in 2010 to 0.81 in 2011 and 0.80 in 2012 per 1000 ventilator days.

Use of the ERA checklist in paper format was inconsistent at the outset of the project implementation. This situation led to some children not having an ERA conducted despite meeting assessment criteria and thus failed extubations. Inconsistent adoption of the paper ERA was attributed to the checklist not being part of the workflow, the culture of belief that failed extubations are acceptable, and unclear role expectations for the RNs and RTs.

Subsequently, the inclusion of the RT educator assisted with RT role definition and adoption of the ERA checklist and protocol. The integration of the ERA into the electronic medical record assisted with the easy use of the ERA because it became part of the workflow. From the initiation of the intubation, through the daily patient assessment and the plan for extubation, the ERA guided the process. Continued education of the PICU RN staff was accomplished through staff huddles and individual sessions, which addressed role expectations. Staff education also included an introduction of the evidence-based process and sharing of current literature findings from the nurse manager.

With the assistance of the physician champion, updates were conducted for the PICU intensivists. The inclusion of the ERA checklist orders at the initiation of intubation assisted with collaboration at the bedside and ERA. Changing the culture from acceptance of reintubations to one of nonacceptance of reintubations was accomplished with the assistance of the physician champion and the PICU medical director. Supporting the culture of collaboration for extubation readiness involved the nurse manager with the team members proactively identifying patients ready for an ERA trail.

RECOMMENDATIONS AND LESSONS LEARNED

The creation of the PICU ERA checklist was accomplished by recognizing and coordinating a multidisciplinary team of stakeholders. Each team member brought a specific skill set and focus that contributed to the overall creation and success of the ERA. Commitment to the team process, such as attending meetings, and fulfilling assigned responsibilities are essential agreements that need to be presented early in the process.

Another lesson learned was to conduct an evaluation of the cultural norms of the PICU as part of the initial assessment survey process. The implementation of the ERA trial revealed a long-standing perception and cultural norm that failed extubations were to be expected and demonstrated proactive mechanical ventilator management from the physician perspective. These perceptions and cultural norms were challenges that needed to be addressed. Sharing current literature that supported the reduction of failed extubations and the potential harms associated with reintubations changed these beliefs and fostered adoption by the physician champion and the medical director of the PICU.

The third lesson learned was the importance of assigning responsibility for staff education and implementation early in the project. Not having someone designated to deliver staff education can be a barrier to the adoption of a new tool. By collaborating with the department-designated educators, staff education for the ERA trial and implementation was eventually accomplished. Team members developed consensus as to who was responsible for staff education and began face-to-face promotion of the ERA trial with department educators. Physician education and follow through was assigned to the physician champion and included promotion of the new practice and performance feedback.

The fourth lesson learned was the value of a trial period to test the appropriateness of the criteria and determine how to fit the ERA assessment into the existing work flow. To better assist the trial period, clarity of roles and expectations of the team members would have improved the introduction of the ERA into the work flow. The team created the ERA to be adapted for the electronic medical record. However, the transition from the paper trial to the electronic medical record was delayed because of the lack of information technology department representatives on the team at the outset. This delay slowed the operationalization of the ERA into the work flow including order entry and documentation of the assessment. Early inclusion of personnel from the information technology department would have enhanced the efficiency and adoption of the ERA.

SUMMARY

The reduction of failed extubations in the PICU from 2.47 per 1000 ventilator days to 0.80 per 1000 ventilator days is attributed to the increased collaboration among care providers, use of the ERA checklist, and implementation of the ERA checklist into the work flow. The resulting protocol can now be used to identify and prepare children with nonchronic conditions for extubation. The inclusion of the ERA into the electronic medical record, the clarification of roles and expectations, and a culture shift related to nonacceptance of failed extubations changed and improved patient care.

The use of an evidence-based practice approach in addressing failed extubations for children without previous lung injury and/or neuromuscular conditions created a model for sustained practice change. Inclusion of multidisciplinary stakeholders in the creation, implementation, and evaluation of the ERA checklist enhanced the evidence-based competencies of team members and contributed to other positive outcomes of the project.

An additional and unexpected benefit of this evidence-based practice project included increased collaboration among care providers that will assist in future evaluation of extubation readiness in children, potentially including those with previous lung disease and/or neuromuscular conditions and new quality improvement initiatives in many other areas of PICU patient care.

REFERENCES

1. Ferguson LP, Walsh BK, Munhall D. A spontaneous breathing trial with pressure support overestimates readiness for extubation in children. Pediatr Crit Care Med 2011;12(6):330–5.
2. Frutos-Vivar F, Esteban A, Apeztequia C, et al. Outcome of reintubated patients after scheduled extubation. J Crit Care 2011;26:502–9.
3. Bittner EA, Schmidt UH. Tracheal reintubation: caused by too much of a good thing? Respir Care 2012;57(10):1687–91.
4. Titler MG, Kleiber C, Steelman V, et al. The Iowa Model of Evidence-based Practice to promote quality care. Crit Care Nurs Clin North Am 2001;13(4):497–509.
5. MacIntyre E. Evidence-based guidelines for weaning and discontinuing ventilatory support: a collective task force facilitated by the American College of Chest Physicians; the American Association for Respiratory Care; and the American College of Critical Care Medicine. Chest 2001;120(6):375S–95S.
6. Newth CJ, Venkataraman S, Wilson DF, et al. Weaning and extubation readiness in pediatric patients. Pediatr Crit Care Med 2009;10(1):1–11.
7. Vankataraman ST, Khan N, Brown A. Validation of predictors of extubation success and failure in mechanically ventilated infants and children. Crit Care Med 2000;28(8):2991–6.
8. Laham JL, Brehemy PJ, Rush A. Do clinical parameters predict first planned extubation outcome in the pediatric intensive care unit? J Intensive Care Med 2013. http://dx.doi.org/10.117/088506661349338.

Shhh… I'm Growing: Noise in the NICU

Vickie Laubach, RNC-NIC, MSN*, Patricia Wilhelm, RNC-NIC, PhD, Katie Carter, RNC-NIC, BSN

KEYWORDS

- Noise • Preterm • Neonatal • Neonatal intensive care unit • Newborns • Infants
- Sound • Sound levels

KEY POINTS

- Attempting to mitigate operational and structural sounds is important in improving the outcomes of high-risk preterm infants.
- It was anticipated that a culture change in nursing behaviors to include "Quiet Time" would result in reducing the noise levels towards the National Recommended Safe Sound Levels.
- Operational and structural changes were also required in order to provide a safer neurophysiological environment for the rest and growth of the neonate and close the gap to achieve National Recommended Safe Sound Levels.

INTRODUCTION

In 2012, nearly 500,000 babies were born preterm (before 37 weeks' gestation) in the United States.[1] Most of these premature neonates will spend the first weeks to months of their lives in the neonatal intensive care unit (NICU). The NICU is often designed as one large room or "Open-Bay" where staff can monitor multiple infants all in one space. This large, open room environment lends itself to persistent and unpredictable sounds that are in stark contrast to the protective environment of a mother's womb. The continuous sounds from cardiopulmonary (CR) monitors, noisy heating and air duct systems, and conversations between staff and family that are commonplace in

Disclosures: None.
Disclaimer: The views expressed in this presentation are those of the author(s) and do not reflect the official policy or position of the Department of the Army, Department of the Defense, or the US government.
Neonatal Intensive Care Unit, Tripler Army Medical Center, 1 Jarrett White Road, MCHK-PE, Honolulu, HI 96859, USA
* Corresponding author.
E-mail address: alaub41324@aol.com

Nurs Clin N Am 49 (2014) 329–344
http://dx.doi.org/10.1016/j.cnur.2014.05.007
0029-6465/14/$ – see front matter Published by Elsevier Inc.

the NICU, increase the risk of hearing loss, and can have a negative impact on neurosensory and physiologic short-term and long-term developmental outcomes for the premature neonate.[2-7] The exposure to operational and structural sounds can result in acute physical and behavioral changes that interrupt the natural growth and development of the neonate.[7]

Attempting to mitigate these potentially harmful sounds is important in improving the outcomes of high-risk preterm infants. An evidence-based nursing guideline for structured "Quiet Time" and education on operational practice changes were established in the Open-Bay NICU to reduce noise levels before the conversion to a Single Family Room (SFR) NICU.[8] It was anticipated that a culture change in nursing behaviors would result from operational changes and NICU renovations. This culture change would lead to a safer neurophysiological environment for the rest and growth of the neonate. The Iowa Model of Evidence-Based Practice to Promote Quality Care was the framework used to guide this evidence-based practice project (**Box 1**).[9]

ORGANIZATIONAL PRIORITY AND FORM A TEAM

A nurse-driven evidence-based practice (EBP) team was formed. The EBP team identified this project as a priority based on the mission, vision, and strategic goals of the NICU and the organization to create improved outcomes for the patient. The team consisted of a NICU physician champion, NICU nurse manager, clinical nurse specialist, staff registered nurses, and an industrial hygienist. The team set out to identify current sound levels in the Open-Bay NICU, identify the recommended safe sound levels, identify causes of excessive sound levels, and implement changes to improve practices on the unit.

EVIDENCE FOR PRACTICE IMPROVEMENT

There have been numerous studies reported over the past 25 years on sound levels in the NICU environment, and the deleterious impact of excessive sound levels on the growth and development of the premature infant. The American Academy of Pediatrics Committee on Environmental Health concluded that sounds levels in the NICU should be maintained at or below 45 dB.[2] The Study Group on Neonatal Intensive Care Unit Sound identified that (1) intrauterine fetus exposure to sound varies greatly from extrauterine exposure, (2) inappropriate sound exposure (consistency, reverberation, frequency, and excessive levels) causes negative neurosensory and physiologic long-term developmental outcomes related to the maturation process, and (3) technology exists for all NICUs to measure and identify causes of inappropriate sound exposure to the neonate.[2,5,6] The Study Group concluded with recommendations for safe sound levels and developmental practices to improve the environmental setting for the neonate in the NICU.

LITERATURE REVIEW

The review of literature was conducted to find research related to (1) consensus of current safe sound level recommendations, (2) noise exposure linked to developmental outcomes, (3) recommended methods of sound measurement, and (4) associated operational and structural causes of noise. Key terms used for the literature search were "noise, preterm, neonatal, neonatal intensive care unit, newborns, infants, sound, and sound levels." The database search engines, Medline, CINAHL, Cochrane, TRIP, Bandolier, National Guideline Clearinghouse, and PubMed were searched for

Box 1
The Iowa model for evidence-based practice to promote quality care

1. Problem-focused and knowledge-focused triggers:

    A. Operational practices

    B. Structural practices

    C. Unknown sound levels in Open-Bay NICU

    D. National Recommended Sound Levels

2. Priority to the organization:

    A. Meets the balanced score card for improving outcomes

3. Form a team:

    A. Nurse-driven team (NICU nurse manager, clinical nurse specialist, staff registered nurses)

    B. Physician champion (NICU director)

    C. Industrial hygienist

4. Assembled relevant research

    A. Key search terms

    B. 65 articles, narrowed to 22 for topic relevance

    C. Critique for evidence

    D. Three guidelines: National Recommended Levels

5. Pilot the change in practice

    A. Baseline sound level data (random ambient, common practices, structural sounds in Open-Bay NICU and simulated SFR to NRL)

    B. Staff education

    C. "Quiet Time" guideline implemented

6. Evaluate process and outcomes

    A. Adopted change in practice

    B. Collected random ambient sound levels in Open-Bay NICU after change in practice

    C. Compared ambient sound levels in Open-Bay NICU, simulated SFR, before and after change in practice compared with NRL

7. Monitor and analyze structure, process, and outcome data

    A. Sound project: supported structural changes for sound-abatement materials for new renovation environment

    B. Sound meter devices implemented in each SFR and hallway for continually monitoring sound levels

    C. Staff and family education for reminders to practices that reduce sound levels in the SFR: sustain the gain of change!

8. Disseminate results

    A. Stakeholders, organization, staff

    B. Similar organizations to create change in practice

Data from Titler MG, Kleiber C, Steelman VJ, et al. The Iowa model of evidence-based practice to promote quality care. Crit Care Nurs Clin North Am 2001;13(4):497–509.

relevant literature. The literature review yielded 65 articles and 3 guidelines dating from 1997 to the time of the EBP project in 2010. Of the 65 articles, the search was narrowed to 15 articles that were relevant to the EBP. Critique for strength of evidence using the Mosby's Level of Evidence[10] and the AGREE tool[11] provided support to drive changes in operational and structural practices within the NICU to promote positive outcomes for the neonate (**Table 1**).

Recommended Safe Sound Levels

The current nationally recognized safe sound levels for the infant rooms in the NICU should not exceed 45 to 50 dB, with transient sound not to exceed 65 to 70 dB. To promote an optimal environment for rest and growth of the neonate, a combination of continuous background and operational sound should be considered.[2,5,10] Gravens[5] concluded that if operational and structural recommendations were followed, the NICU environment would promote positive growth, increase physiologic stability, increase neurosensory development, facilitate bonding, and reduce potential long-term adverse effects on speech and auditory development.

Noise Exposure Linked to Developmental Outcomes

Johnson found that increased environmental sound is a cause of stress for the neonate, which leads to agitation and increased morbidity.[12,13] Adverse physiologic effects of noise on the preterm infant included increased blood pressure, heart rate, respiratory rate, and decreased oxygen saturation; thus, stress from increased noise levels caused an increased need in oxygen and caloric consumption.[4,14,15] Events of acute distress in response to increased noise levels can lead to life-threatening situations, such as sudden and severe decrease in oxygen saturation, as well as apneic and bradycardia events.[3,4]

Methods of Sound Level Measurement

There was no specific length of time that was considered a golden standard to measure the sound levels in the NICU. Several articles found that overall sound levels varied in relation to the unit staff activities, time of day or night, day of the week, patient acuity, equipment, and the level of the NICU (Mosby Level I, II, III). Sound measurements were conducted over 2 hours and up to 24 hours, on 1 day versus 9 days, or 1 day every week for 1 year.[4,14–21] At the time of this EBP project in the Open-Bay

Table 1		
Levels of evidence: literature review		
Mosby's Level	**Description**	**No. of Articles on Sound Levels in the Neonatal Intensive Care Unit**
Level I	Meta-analysis	—
Level II	Experimental design (randomized controlled trial)	—
Level III	Quasi-experimental design	3
Level IV	Case controlled, cohort study	1
Level V	Correlation studies	2
Level VI	Descriptive or qualitative design	9
Level VII	Authority opinion or expert committee report	3

Key search terms were noise, Preterm, Neonatal, Neonatal Intensive Care Unit, Newborns, Infants, sound, and sound Levels.

NICU, the ambient sound levels were unknown, practitioners were unaware of recommended guidelines for safe sound levels, and there were no sound measurement devices used in the NICU to alert staff of excessive sound levels. Staff was unaware of the specific operational practices and structural nuances that lend to excessive and obtrusive sound levels that can cause negative neurophysical short-term and long-term outcomes for the developing neonate.

Associated Operational and Structural Causes of Noise

Operational causes of noise can be changed through education, change in care practices, and modification of procedures.[22] Noise also can be affected by the overall structural environment of the unit. For example, metal trash cans are louder than plastic trash cans, and ceiling tiles and flooring tiles have different sound ratings that mitigate noise.[13–16] Operational changes and nursing practice behavior changes may have the greatest impact on lowering sound levels. These also may be the least-expensive changes to make but may be the most challenging to implement and sustain.[4,18] Overcoming obstacles associated with achieving safe sound levels requires an awareness and buy-in of the multidisciplinary staff to honor and adopt a change in culture to create a safe sound environment for the neonate.

IMPLEMENTATION STRATEGIES
Outcomes to Be Achieved

The goal was to achieve the National Recommended Safe Sound Level (NRL) of 45 to 50 dB in a Level III NICU at a tertiary care center. The objectives of this EBP project were to (1) identify staff perceptions of current sound levels in the NICU, (2) measure current sound levels (ambient, impact, and continuous) in an Open-Bay Level III NICU and simulated SFR, (3) determine if the sound levels met the NRL, (4) identify and implement changes in practice to support sound levels consistent with the NRL before renovation, and finally (5) measure the sound levels in the newly renovated SFR NICU and compare with the NRL.

Project: Phase 1, Baseline Data

The first phase involved 4 steps: (1) survey staff regarding their perceptions of noise in the NICU, (2) measure continuous and impact levels of operational sound on the ambient environment of the infant, (3) obtain random continuous sound levels in the Open-Bay NICU in 3 of the 4 patient-care pods (18-bed Open-Bay NICU covering 3300 square feet) as well as in a simulated SFR, and (4) obtain ambient sound levels in the SFR NICU.

Step 1

The Staff Survey was distributed to gather baseline information on the multidisciplinary staff perception of sound levels in the NICU, current knowledge of potential effects of excessive sound levels on the neonate, and identify gaps in knowledge (**Box 2**). Thirty-eight qualitative anonymous surveys were distributed with 31 returned responses (82% return rate) from staff nurses, neonatologists, and other ancillary staff (unit desk clerk, respiratory therapist, pharmacist, and lactation consultant (**Table 2**)).

Step 2

The mean ambient sound level was recorded in decibels for a specific time period to gather a baseline sound level in the Open-Bay NICU before implementation of education or changes in practice. The baseline random ambient sound levels were obtained in the Open-Bay NICU over a period of time during the day shift in Pods 1, 2, and 3. The

---

Box 2
Staff survey

Specify your role in the unit: nurse/physician/respiratory technician/other

Questions:

1. What time of the day or night do you think is the noisiest on the unit?

2. What location on the unit do you think is the noisiest?

3. What care practices/activities do you think create the most noise?

4. What effects do you think that noise levels have on the health of the infant?

5. What do you think this unit has done to address noise levels?

6. Tell me what change could be made on the unit to positively affect noise levels?

7. Do you think implementing a "Quiet Time" would affect noise levels on the unit?

---

data were collected in average and peak decibel readings and reported as a mean ambient sound level for the time period. There was no control over the census or acuity at the time of data collection, as the NICU is a dynamic environment that inherently experiences constant change in census, acuity, and number of staff or visitors (**Fig. 1**).

Ambient sound levels were obtained and recorded from both inside and outside of the isolette. Some high-risk infants are cared for on radiant warmers or open cribs and do not have the protection or sound abatement provided by the double-wall isolette while in the NICU and are therefore subjected to the same sound as the adults within the environment. Impact and continuous sounds were produced by replicating a sound 10 times; that is, opening and closing doors, writing on the isolette top, or dropping a heavy item into the metal garbage can next to the infant bedside. Sound levels were then measured and recorded in mean decibels. Continuous sound, as determined by the industrial hygienists, was measured as a range of sound with lowest and highest values recorded and expressed as a mean. A list of 46 specific operational practices and structural sounds were identified as potential noise in the NICU and 27 of the most common were measured. A convenience sampling was used because not all practices could practicably be recorded due to the lack of availability of the equipment in the unit at the time of data collection. The sounds were recorded as the events occurred (eg, pneumatic tube system, ringing phones, and CR alarms) to evaluate the sound levels as they occur normally and randomly in the NICU environment.

Continuous ambient sound levels were measured by a sound meter in decibels, in 3 pods of the NICU over random 2-hour to 24-hour time periods on 10 random days from November 2009 to September 2011. The dosimeter sound meter used for prerenovation sound measurement was a handheld or mounted data logger with a microphone that measured both continuous and impact sound levels over a specified time frame. An environmental industrial hygienist engineer from the facility was consulted regarding the project, how to obtain and analyze the data, and where to locate the meters during random ambient data collection in the open-bay pods to ensure nonobstructive readings. The dosimeter was calibrated by the sound meter manufacturing experts before obtaining sound levels and periodically throughout the project to ensure reliability and validity of the equipment. Data were collected and recorded as a value per minute and then reported as an average decibel value per hour (**Fig. 2**).

Step 3
A simulated SFR was equipped with an isolette, metal garbage can, metal hamper, and various supplies or equipment that the staff would use for care practices.

Table 2 Staff survey results (October 2009)	
Comments/Responses	Percentage
Time of day or night the noisiest?	
1. Day	45
2. Night	8
3. Shift change at 0600 and 1800 daily	47
Location in NICU the noisiest?	
1. Front or entrance of the NICU	68
2. Charge nurse and physician desk areas	32
Staff perceptions: care practices/activities create the most noise?	
1. Shift reports and multidisciplinary rounds	58
2. General conversation/visitors, families, siblings	29
3. Other: monitors and alarms	13
What effects noise levels have on health of infant?	
1. Physiologic (HR, BP, O_2 or saturation changes)	32
2. Brain development affected	32
3. Agitation/stress	19
4. Sleep interruptions	17
What has the NICU done to address noise levels?	
1. Nothing	39
2. Verbal reminders, silence alarms: operational change	50
3. Plan to redesign unit: structural change	11
Staff perceptions: What change could be made to positively affect noise levels?	
1. Noise monitor	29
2. Response to alarms, phones, lower voices, dim lights	52
3. Single family room design	10
4. Other (education, close unit for shift change)	9
Would implementation of "Quiet Time" reduce sound levels?	
1. Yes	55
2. No	13
3. Maybe/Unsure	32

Response rate: (n = 31) 82%.
Abbreviations: BP, blood pressure; HR, heart rate; NICU, neonatal intensive care unit.

Operational sounds are those practices staff has the ability to control and change to reduce sound levels in the NICU. Continuous and impact sound levels were measured and recorded in average mean decibel levels. Sound levels were obtained in this environment to control the extraneous sounds to gather data only on operational sounds (**Fig. 3**).

Step 4
The newly renovated SFR NICU was equipped with sound-monitoring devices placed within each patient room. A sound-monitoring device is designed to alert staff to excessive noise based on a color change from green to yellow to red based on alert levels that were set to meet NRL. A green light indicates noise is within the NRL. A yellow light indicates that the noise is starting to exceed NRL, and red indicates that the level exceeds NRL and actions must be taken to decrease the noise. An empty room

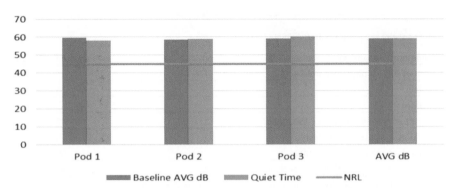

Fig. 1. Baseline random ambient sound levels in the Open-Bay NICU.

close to the front entrance was set up to include a prewarming isolette and equipment that would be used on admission of any infant. Sound data in decibels were downloaded from the device (**Fig. 4**).

In addition, 3 SFRs occupied with infant(s) were chosen at random on 3 separate days and data were pulled over a 24-hour period of time. Continuous sound levels were averaged over the 24-hour period in decibels (**Fig. 5**).

Project: Phase 2, Developing and Implementing the Guideline

The second phase included (1) analyzing the data obtained from the multidisciplinary staff survey, (2) displaying the continuous and impact sound levels of operational practices and comparing them with the NRL, (3) developing and implementing an education module based on gaps in knowledge about sound level findings compared with NRL, (4) developing and implementing a "Quiet Time Guideline," and (5) implementing operational and structural changes to reduce causes of excessive sound levels in the NICU with the SFR renovation.

Staff identified day shift (0900–1100) during multidisciplinary rounds and shift change (0600 and 1800) as times of increased noise levels. The entrance area of

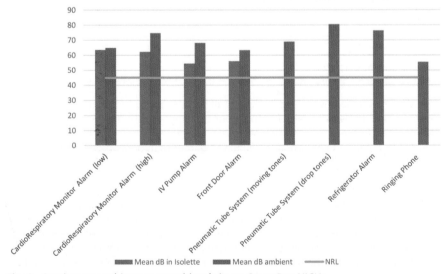

Fig. 2. Continuous and impact sound levels in an Open-Bay NICU.

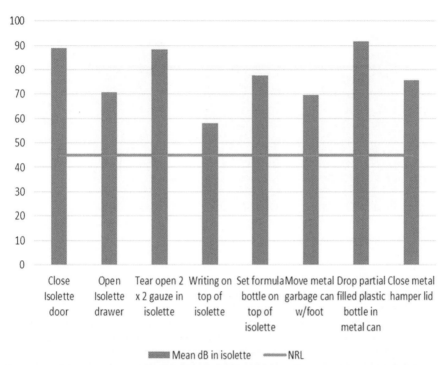

Fig. 3. Continuous and impact sound levels from operational practices in a simulated SFR.

the NICU was the noisiest because of the ringing of phones, the pneumatic tube system, influx of visitors and ancillary support staff, and common congregation of staff. The staff identified operational practices that increased noise levels, such as loud general socializing conversations among staff and families, and not silencing alarms quickly were commonplace in the Open-Bay environment. Staff observed anecdotally that neonates exposed to excess sound levels experience agitation, stress,

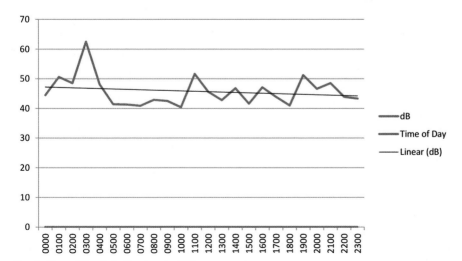

Fig. 4. Sound levels in the empty SFR.

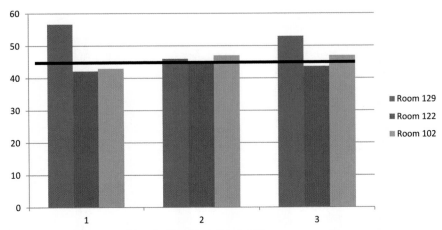

Fig. 5. SFR ambient sound levels. The *black line* is NRL.

interference with sleep, increased heart rate, overstimulation, and fluctuations in blood pressure and oxygen saturations within the Open-Bay NICU.

The baseline average random ambient sound levels in the Open-Bay NICU, Pods 1, 2, and 3, revealed that the baseline was 58 to 60 dB. All 3 Pods were loud and exceeded the NRL. Pod 1 was the loudest at 60 dB and was located closest to the alarm on the front door, the pneumatic tube system, and the physician's work area.

Impact and continuous sounds ranged from 55.5 dB inside the isolette to as high as 80.5 dB from the pneumatic tube system when a tube was arriving into the NICU at the front desk area near Pod 1. All continuous and impact sounds measured as both ambient and within the isolette exceeded the NRL.

In the simulated SFR, continuous and impact sound levels ranged from 57.6 dB to as high as 101.4 dB when closing the door of the isolette. When moving the metal trash can across the room with a foot, a common infection-control practice, sound levels ranged from 64.9 dB to 71.9 dB inside the infant's isolette. Whisper or quiet conversation in a simulated environment was noted to meet the NRL at 30 dB. However, most continuous and impact sounds that were generated from operational practices in a simulated SFR environment without structural noise reduction changes still exceeded NRL.

Before the renovation to the SFR NICU, an education module was developed and administered to the multidisciplinary staff on the effects and outcomes associated with excessive noise on the neonate. The education module consisted of providing knowledge on the NRL compared with current sound levels in the Open-Bay NICU, sound levels associated with common day-to-day operational care practices, and survey results. The purpose of this education was to close the knowledge gap, and to create buy-in and ownership by staff to facilitate change in care practice. Changes in operational care practices were emphasized to create a culture of behavior change, and structural changes were implemented for sound abatement for the renovation of the SFR NICU.

Quiet Time Guidelines

A guideline was developed and a daily "Quiet Time" was implemented in the Open-Bay NICU from 1430 to 1530. The goal was to institute change in practice before moving into the SFR environment. The SFRs would expand the footprint from the

3300-square-foot Open-Bay 20-bed NICU to a 22-bed SFR NICU spanning over approximately 10,000 square feet.

Open-Bay NICU

The "Quiet Time" guideline included dimmed lights, noise levels to be kept at a minimum, and conversation encouraged at whisper tones (**Fig. 6**).

Visitors were allowed to visit; however, they were expected to abide by the Quiet Time guidelines. Parents were educated and engaged as a part of the team to foster a family-centered care model. To ensure quiet time was followed, parents were encouraged to arrive early to settle in with kangaroo care before the scheduled Quiet Time. The charge registered nurse and/or ward clerk were responsible for posting signage at all door entrances and alerting the staff of Quiet Time. Patient-care activities were completed either before or after the Quiet Time, unless an emergent situation occurred that would preclude the Quiet Time on that day.

SFRs

The renovation to a 22-bed SFR process took almost 3 years from start to finish. Half of the unit was completed in April 2012, and the entire unit was completed in February 2013. Noise-reduction features were integrated into the design from the flooring to the

QUIET TIME GUIDELINES:

* 1430 – 1530 Daily

* Reduces noise

* Promotes rest & healing

* Fosters:
  Family Centered Care
  Developmental Care

* Supports mission & vision of TAMC NICU Ohana

NICU Ohana's

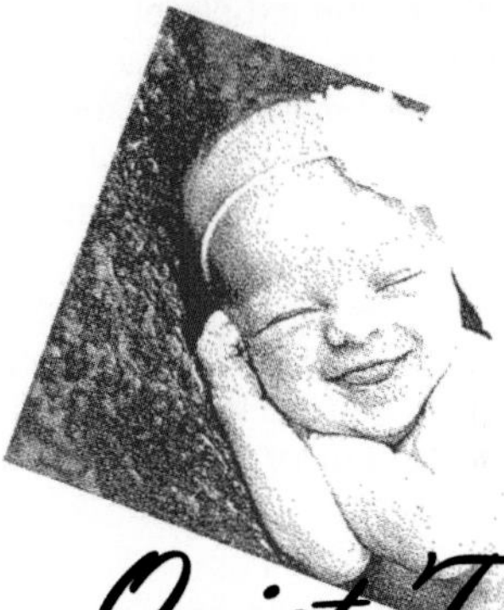

Quiet Time

We ask for your kokua in helping us provide a Quiet Time from 1430 to 1530 daily, which allows our babies an opportunity for rest time.

During this time we will have the lights dimmed. This is a minimal handling and minimal stimulation time period. Only essential activities and personnel will be allowed in the unit at this time. Moms, dads, and visitors are welcome.

We ask for quiet, whisper voices so our babies can sleep and grow!

If you have any questions, please ask one of our NICU staff members.

Fig. 6. Quiet Time guidelines.

ceiling tile. Once patients were cared for in the SFRs, the sound meters provided continuous monitoring of sound levels.

EVALUATION

Random and continuous ambient and impact sound levels were measured before and after implementation of evidence-based practice changes in the Open-Bay NICU before the renovation to an SFR. Additional continuous ambient sound levels were obtained from the SFR NICU after renovation. The data provided insight on the sound levels that the neonate is exposed to throughout the time they are in the NICU. After baseline data collection, education, and dissemination of results to the staff on how to reduce or eliminate the excessive noise levels, a designated Quiet Time guideline was implemented to secure time for the rest and healing of the neonate. After the implementation of the designated Quiet Time, random ambient sound levels were obtained to measure the effectiveness of having a designated Quiet Time. These sound levels were compared with baseline and NRL (**Fig. 7**).

Although the staff received education to increase knowledge and awareness of the effects of sound associated with daily common operational practices on the developing neonate, it was discovered that constant gentle reminders were needed to keep staff compliant and promote change in practice to reduce the sound levels in the Open-Bay NICU. Visual reminders, such as signage or seeing the sound meter in the unit, also motivated the multidisciplinary staff to adhere to the practice. These sounds, operational and structural, all exceeded the NRLs in the Open-Bay unit.

The SFR NICU with added structural sound abatement design features and the visual light reminder have brought the sound levels closer to the NRL. The average decibel level in the SFR over a 24-hour period was 46.32 dB. Although slightly exceeding the NRL, it was considerably lower than the 57.6 dB from the simulated SFR (**Fig. 8**).

Three SFRs were randomly selected on 3 different days while occupied by infant(s). The data were analyzed and mean decibel levels were calculated over a 24-hour period. The ambient sound levels ranged from 42.13 dB to 56.69 dB, demonstrating that it is possible to care for infants in a room and maintain the sound levels at or below

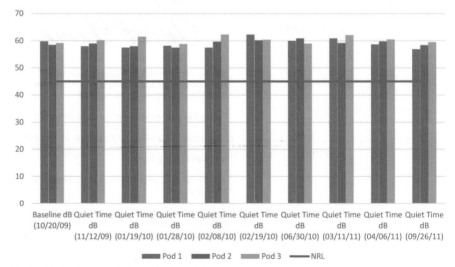

Fig. 7. Ambient sound levels during Quiet Time.

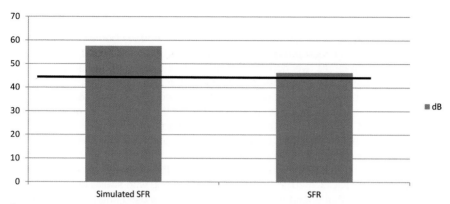

Fig. 8. Comparison levels of the simulated SFR and the SFR to the NRL. The *black line* is NRL.

the NRL. Any additional equipment that was placed in the room (ie, ventilators or oscillators) added additional continuous noise. Critical infants, who require these additional pieces of equipment, are generally cared for in one of the larger SFRs that often had the highest sound levels. When comparing the SFR ambient sound levels to the Open-Bay NICU levels, it is clear that the structural modifications with the renovation were effective in closing the gap to achieve the NRL. Of the 9 measured days in 3 occupied SFRs, the mean sound levels were at or below the NRL on 4 days (44%). However, there are still transient times when there are brief increases in sound levels due to operational practices, conversations, and equipment.

Parents play an important role in helping to monitor and secure an environment that supports the growth and development of their newborn. Parents are educated on admission to the SFR and the operational practices (ie, whisper voices, cell phones to vibrate) and the sound device that helps to visually alert if the NRL is exceeded. Parents are empowered as valued members of the team.

LESSONS LEARNED

Creating change in behavior associated with care practice takes time and commitment by all members of the staff. Although several operational care practices and structural changes were identified and implemented to reduce the noise levels in the Open-Bay NICU to meet the NRL, only a slight reduction was appreciated within this environment. The conversion to the SFR NICU with additional structural changes resulted in an overall reduction in sound levels and closed the gap to meet the NRL. It is possible to achieve sound levels at or below the NRL. It can be done.

However, the gap still exists and there is a continued need to reinforce operational care practices to meet the NRL all the time. Ongoing education on the effects of sound, changes in operational care practices to reduce exposure to excessive sound levels, along with gentle reminders, such as posted signage, securing a designated Quiet Time and monitoring sound levels continuously or intermittently, should be a routine practice regardless of the design of the NICU. Eliminating equipment such as metal trash cans, linen carts, hampers, and ringing phones are other cost-effective ways to reduce sound levels should a full renovation not be feasible. Engaging parents as members of the team remains key to sustainability. Providing education on sound reduction, encouraging quiet whisper voices, securing quiet time with their newborn, alerting staff of visual sound-monitoring cues, and silencing cell phones are other EBPs to reduce harmful noise in the NICU.

RECOMMENDATIONS

It is clear that the renovation to an SFR NICU has tremendous benefits for the developmental growth and neuroprotection of the neonate. Loud noise can be harmful, and therefore any measures we can take to alleviate noxious stimuli is appreciated. Despite the beneficial improvements brought on through renovation, there is still a need to respect the environment of the developing neonate. The use of noise meters to continually monitor the noise is key to maintaining the sound levels at or below the NRL. The visual reminders are helpful during periods of increased activity at the bedside and, even if renovation is not feasible, the purchase of sound meters with visual cues could potentially make a lasting impact.

Structural sound levels were addressed through the complete renovation of the Open-Bay to SFR NICU in 2012. This EBP project, along with sound data, supported changes to ensure that sound abatement materials were used and the overall design focused on decreasing exposure of noise to the neonate. Sound abatement materials with high ratings of sound absorption, such as flooring and ceiling tiles designed to reduce noise, were installed in the SFR. The sound abatement materials were critical components to achieving the NRL.

The SFR design created a decentralization to reduce socialization and congregation of staff. Nurses who once congregated at the nurses' station are now located closer to the bedside with individual charting stations available for documentation and observation of their individual infant assignment. Multidisciplinary rounds once conducted at the infants' bedside in the Open-Bay are now conducted outside of the infants' SFR followed by personal rounds with individual families in whispered tones. The breast milk freezer, pneumatic tube system, linen cart, and door alarms were placed away from the patient-care areas.

Significant collaboration among the alarm systems engineers, industrial hygienist, and leadership enabled the setting of the fire alarms, infant abduction alarms, and code alarms to fall within safety standards and remain as close to the NRL as possible. In addition, keeping in mind the safety standards, critical infant alarms were selected based on specific criteria, which prevented nuisance alarms from contributing to excessive sound levels and the alarm volume from the monitor is set to alert staff at an appropriate level. Alarms transmitted to the handheld devices, carried by the staff, also were set at a preselected volume level. Wall phones in the SFR have no ring tone and are signaled by flashing lights. Metal garbage cans and linen hampers were replaced with plastic.

Sound meters have been installed in all SFRs for continuous monitoring with visual reminders to encourage staff and visitors to keep conversations within the NRL standards. Sound measurements are monitored and recorded continuously via a sound meter device that has been installed in each SFR and both common hallways. The continuous monitoring device is programed for a specific decibel level so that when the threshold has been reached, a visible light warning creates a cue to staff, parents, and visitors that the sound levels are to be decreased to support a more developmentally appropriate environment for the infant.

Education on the sound meter is provided to all incoming staff. Education also is provided as an integral part of the parent orientation to their infant's room and developmental environment on admission to the NICU. This ensures a team approach and collaboration among the family and staff to create a culture of safety for the infant. Sound data are recorded continuously and can be analyzed and compared with NRL at any given time.

In the SFR NICU, there are no longer 1-hour periods of Quiet Time each day. Quiet Time is all the time and not a specific designated time because the SFR physical environment supports this practice for each individual patient and as a whole for the unit. The SFR design and increasing staff knowledge through education has allowed for individualizing a neuroprotective environment for the neonate to promote quality outcomes through EBP.

SUMMARY

Not every NICU will have the opportunity to participate in a total renovation to assist in the goal toward achieving NRL. However, there are several simple yet cost-effective measures, for example, replacing metal trash cans with plastic ones, turning pagers to vibrate rather than ring, turning down the volume of phones, and installing 1 or 2 sound meters, that can be taken to reduce the sounds that impact the growth and development of the premature infant. These operational practices and structural changes that have been recommended along with continuously monitoring the infants' environment can reduce sound levels within the NICU. The implementation of a Quiet Time guideline for extended periods was instrumental to achieving the NRL. Despite renovation to the SFR NICU, there continues to be a need to reinforce operational practices that impact the sound levels. Sound levels above the NRL will continue to be a challenge when caring for infants in the NICU; however, this evidence-based practice project demonstrated that simple changes can make a difference in sound exposure in the neonate population.

ACKNOWLEDGMENTS

The authors acknowledge the Hawaii State Center for Nursing for their support of this project.

REFERENCES

1. Centers for Disease Control and Prevention. FastStats. 2013. Available at: http://www.cdc.gov/nchs/fastats/birthwt.htm. Accessed August 6, 2013.
2. Noise: a hazard for the fetus and newborn. American Academy of Pediatrics, Committee on Environmental Health. Pediatrics 1997;100(4):724–7.
3. Bremmer P, Byers JF, Kiehl E. Noise and the premature infant: physiological effects and practice implications. J Obstet Gynecol Neonatal Nurs 2003;32(4): 447–53.
4. Darcy AE, Hancock LE, Ware EJ. A descriptive study of noise in the neonatal intensive care unit: ambient levels and perceptions of contributing factors. Adv Neonatal Care 2008;8(Suppl 5):S16–26.
5. Gravens SN. The full-term and premature newborn: sound and the developing infant in the NICU: conclusions and recommendations for care. J Perinatol 2000;20: S88–93.
6. Consensus Committee on Recommending Design Standards for Advanced Neonatal Care (RSCCNICUD). Recommended standards for newborn ICU design. 2007.
7. VandenBerg KA. Individualized developmental care for high risk newborns in the NICU: a practice guideline. Early Hum Dev 2007;83:433–42.
8. Zwick MB. Decreasing environmental noise in the NICU through staff education. Neonatal Intensive Care 1993;6(2):16–9.
9. Titler MG, Kleiber C, Steelman VJ, et al. The Iowa model of evidence-based practice to promote quality care. Crit Care Nurs Clin North Am 2001;13(4): 497–509.

10. The Mosby's levels of evidence are: a focus on adult acute and critical care. Worldviews Evid Based Nurs 2004;1(3):194–7 Adapted from Melnyk BM. (2004); modified from Guyatt&Rennie (2002), Harris et al. (2001).

11. Cluzeau FA, Burgers JS, Brouwers JS, et al. AGREE collaboration: development and validation of an international appraisal instrument for assessing the quality of clinical practice guidelines: the AGREE project. Qual Saf Health Care 2003;12(1): 18–23.

12. Johnson AN. Neonatal response to control of noise inside the incubator. Pediatr Nurs 2001;27(6):600–5.

13. Johnson AN. Adapting the neonatal intensive care environment to decrease noise. J Perinat Neonatal Nurs 2003;17(4):280–8.

14. Byers JF, Waugh WR, Lowman LB. Sound level exposure of high-risk infants in different environmental conditions. Neonatal Netw 2006;25(1):25–32.

15. Thomas KA, Uran A. How the NICU environment sounds to a preterm infant: update. MCN Am J Matern Child Nurs 2007;32(4):250–3.

16. Brandon DH, Ryan DJ, Barnes AH. Effect of environmental changes on noise in the NICU. Neonatal Netw 2008;26(4):213–7.

17. Krueger C, Schue S, Parker L. Neonatal intensive care unit sound levels before and after structural reconstruction. MCN Am J Matern Child Nurs 2007;32(6): 358–62.

18. Levy GD, Woolston DJ, Browne JV. Mean noise amounts in level II vs level III Neonatal Intensive Care Units. Neonatal Netw 2003;22(2):33–8.

19. Lasky RE, Williams AL. Noise and light exposures for extremely low birth weight newborns during their stay in the neonatal intensive care unit. Pediatrics 2009; 123(2):540–6.

20. Gray L, Philbin K. The acoustic environment of hospital nurseries: measuring sound in hospital nurseries. J Perinatol 2000;20:S99–103.

21. Kellam B, Bhatia J. Sound spectral analysis in the intensive care nursery: measuring high-frequency sound. J Pediatr Nurs 2008;23(4):317–23.

22. DePaul D, Chambers SE. Environmental noise in the neonatal intensive care unit: implications for nursing practice. J Perinat Neonatal Nurs 1995;8(4):71–6.

Evidence-Based Practice for Pain Identification in Cognitively Impaired Nursing Home Residents

Christina Sacoco, RN, MS*, Sally Ishikawa, RN, NHA, MPH, C-DONA

KEYWORDS

- Pain assessment in cognitively impaired elderly residents • Nursing home facility
- Long-term care facility

KEY POINTS

- Pain identification of cognitively impaired elderly is very challenging.
- There is a crucial need for recognizing pain in nursing home residents because it is often underreported in skilled nursing facilities and long-term care facilities.
- A project carried out by nurses in a Hawaii state LTC facility identified a best practice for assessing pain in this particular population.

INTRODUCTION

The quality of nursing care in skilled nursing facilities (SNFs) is overseen by both federal and state agencies. Federally, the Medicare Conditions of Participation, Conditions for Coverage, and Requirements for SNFs and long-term care (LTC) facilities are sets of requirements for acceptable quality in the operation of health care entities. In addition to each Condition (or Requirement for SNFs and LTC facilities), there is a group of related quality standards that are required to be met. Compliance with these quality standards is assessed by State survey agencies. The Interpretive Guidelines serve to interpret and clarify the Conditions or Requirements for SNFs and LTC facilities, which define or explain the relevant statute and regulations. Deficiencies are based on a violation of the statute or regulations, which, in turn, are based on observations of the provider's performance or practices.[1]

Disclosures: None.
This project was partially funded by the Agency for Healthcare Research & Quality, 5R13HS017892; Hawaii State Center for Nursing; and Queen Emma Nursing Institute, The Queen's Medical Center, Honolulu, HI.
Leahi Hospital, 3675 Kilauea Avenue, Honolulu, HI 96816, USA
* Corresponding author.
E-mail address: csacoco@hhsc.org

In April 2009, the Centers for Medicare and Medicaid Services (CMS) revised the Interpretive Guidelines for the survey deficiency tag F309, Quality of Care, which states that SNFs and LTC facilities must assess and address pain in all residents, including residents with cognitive impairments.[1] A Core Team of nurse managers in a Hawaii state LTC facility identified the need to improve internal nursing practices relating to pain assessment to meet compliance with the new quality standards. This facility, located in urban Honolulu, Hawaii, is a public 179 bed Medicare dual-certified SNF and Intermediate Care Facility (ICF) and also has 9 acute care beds for inpatient tuberculosis care. The Core Team included Unit Managers, Nursing Supervisors, Resident Assessment Coordinators, the Quality Assurance Coordinator, the Infection Control Coordinator, and the Director of Nursing/Chief Nurse Executive. Specifically, the following nursing practice needs were identified: (1) to improve current pain assessment tools, elevate the level of staff education in pain assessment, and promote awareness of accurately assessing pain; (2) to use a consistent pain assessment tool; and (3) to document pain in residents with cognitive impairment or who lack the ability to communicate the presence of pain to caregivers. The revised CMS guidance standard identified the need to improve overall pain assessment and documentation for all residents. The purpose of this article is to describe the process used to seek the best evidence-based practice (EBP) for pain identification in cognitively impaired nursing home residents and to discuss how the change in practice was implemented at this facility.

EVIDENCE FOR PRACTICE IMPROVEMENT

Among the quality measures (QMs) reported for all nursing homes in the nation, there are 2 categories where the measurement of pain is captured: (1) short stay, which is equal or less than 100 days and (2) long stay, which is equal or greater than 101 days. These QMs are derived from the Minimum Data Set (MDS) of all residents assessed over a given period of time. The MDS is part of the US federally mandated process for clinical assessment of all residents in Medicare- or Medicaid-certified nursing homes, and the MDS is a comprehensive assessment of each resident's functional capabilities that assists nursing home staff to identify individual health problems and needs of residents.[2]

Fig. 1 shows that although this facility scored at or below national and state chronic QM rates for the long-stay residents who have moderate to severe pain as coded on their MDS during 2008 and 2009, this QM was an area in which further internal process improvements could still be made.

Fig. 2 shows the rates for short-stay residents admitted to this facility, who primarily required further rehabilitation following hospitalization for services such as physical, occupational, and/or speech therapy. The rates in October through December 2009 show a slight to moderate increase compared with 2008; however, this represents the decline in the total amount of residents admitted for short-term care during that reporting period.

There is a crucial need for recognizing pain in nursing home residents because it is often underreported in SNFs and LTC facilities. Pain is a common problem for the elderly, especially in the frail older adult who may experience discomfort from common chronic conditions affecting the musculoskeletal system such as arthritis.[3] Nursing home residents with cognitive impairments have high rates of unreported pain when carefully questioned and observed.[4] Nurses are the key to effective pain management; however, studies have demonstrated that nurses lack pain knowledge necessary to manage their residents' pain effectively.[5]

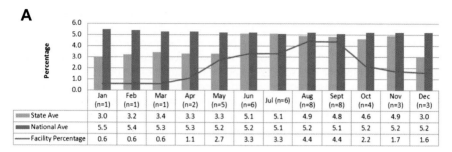

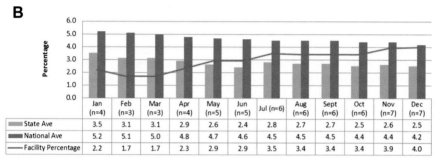

Fig. 1. (*A*) Long-stay residents with moderate to severe pain (2008). (*B*) Long-stay residents with moderate to severe pain (2009).

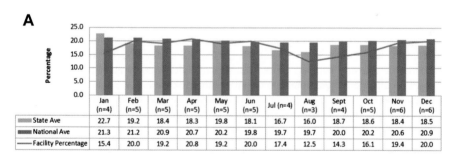

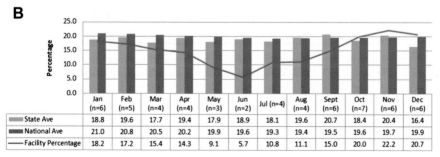

Fig. 2. (*A*) Short-stay residents with moderate to severe pain (2008). (*B*) Short-stay residents with moderate to severe pain (2009).

To determine nursing staff's understanding of the current pain management policies and procedures, as well as the use of pain assessment documentation tools in place at this facility, 33 staff Registered Nurses (RNs) and Licensed Practical Nurses (LPNs) participated in an internally developed written survey, called the Pain Assessment Tool Evaluation Monitor. The tool asked about the extent of the nurse's understanding of the current pain assessment forms and procedures in use. The results of the survey as noted in **Table 1** indicated that the current pain assessment tools, Doloplus-2[6] and the Wong-Baker faces scale,[7] used for cognitively impaired residents were difficult to understand for more than half of the staff nurses.

In October 2009, the Core Team conducted a retrospective chart audit of 27 residents identified as having cognitive impairments (**Table 2**). The audit showed that of the 27 cognitively impaired residents identified with pain symptoms on the MDS, none had comprehensive pain assessment documentation completed. Furthermore, 22% of these residents were reported to have pain symptoms on a daily basis.

As noted in **Fig. 3**, all of the residents identified with pain symptoms had medications ordered for pain; however, only 70% had the cause of pain identified with care plans in place. Of those who had care plans addressing pain, only 35% had nondrug interventions, and only 10% identified the pain scale tool to use to ensure assessment consistency.

Challenges to successfully evaluating and managing pain may include communication difficulties due to illness, language and/or cultural barriers, stoicism about pain, and cognitive impairment.[8–10] The results of the baseline data led the Core Team to analyze the demographic profile of residents as well as staff ethnic composition (**Fig. 4**). It was confirmed that Japanese was the dominant resident ethnicity at 54%. Dominant ethnicity of all staff was Filipino (52%) with 72% of licensed nurses (RNs and LPNs) being of Filipino ethnicity. This mismatch between staff and patient ethnicity further motivated an approach to educate the staff about cultural awareness in the communication and management of pain and to provide appropriate learning tools for the nursing staff.

The Core Team conducted a thorough literature review of all available pain assessment guidelines specific to cognitively impaired residents using Medline and CINAHL databases. Key words used to search for literature included "pain assessment in cognitively impaired residents". The Appraisal of Guidelines for Research & Evaluation (AGREE) instrument[11] was used to critique each guideline.

In addition to the critique results of pain assessment guidelines, the Core Team met to discuss the potential organizational-specific impact that each guideline might present during implementation. Of concern was the use of current pain assessment

Table 1 Leahi Hospital staff nurse survey results of pain tool evaluation (September 2009)	
Comments/Responses	Percentage (%)
Questions how to use the pain assessment form	45
Current pain assessment tools are not easy to use	53
Vital sign flowsheet is used to document pain at least once every 3–6 mo	42
The "Faces" tool is only used when evaluating pain in cognitively impaired residents	67
Reassesses using the appropriate pain assessment tool ("Faces" vs the cognitively impaired pain assessment tool) on a weekly basis until pain is controlled	58
States only the resident defines the goal for pain management	52

Table 2
Leahi Hospital chart audit results of cognitively impaired residents who were coded for pain symptoms on the MDS (N = 27), (October 2009)

Criteria	Percentage (%)
Comprehensive pain assessment completed	0
Pain Symptoms present in a 7-d period:	
Less than daily	78
Daily	22
Mild (eg, pain score 1–3)	78
Moderate (eg, score 4–6)	22
Severe (eg, score 7–10)	0

instruments such as the Doloplus-2 and the Wong-Baker pain scales. Based on the analysis of the literature and in consultation with other interdisciplinary team (IDT) members of the hospital, there was adequate evidence to select and implement the Pain Assessment in Advanced Dementia (PAINAD) assessment tool for the cognitively impaired and nonverbal elders.[12] Key information that the Core Team considered were criteria and associated indicators (based on measurement theory and geriatric pain literature) used in the evaluation of tools for assessing pain in nonverbal elders. PAINAD had the highest score out of 17 pain tools on "The Comparison Grid of Pain Assessment Tools for Non-verbal Older Adults Rated on Evaluation Criteria" score card. Each tool was rated for evidence that supported the criteria and indicators as defined using a 4-point scale.[13]

According to the facility's baseline chart audit results, it was apparent that a pain flowsheet needed to be developed to provide a consistent way for the facility to document and track a resident's pain and effectiveness of the pain management care plan.[14] Furthermore, the team's collaborative efforts established a formalized system-wide interdisciplinary approach to pain management.[14] This approach prompted the Core Team to approach other interdisciplinary members to organize a larger project team to become involved with this facility-wide initiative. Members of this interdisciplinary project team included the Assistant Administrator, Geriatric Psychiatrist, Medical Director, Dietitian, Physical Therapist, Occupational Therapist, Pharmacist, Education Director, Activity Coordinator, Certified Nurse Aides (CNAs), as well as the Core Team members.

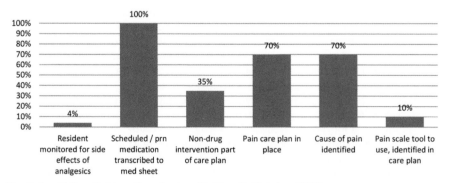

Fig. 3. Leahi Hospital baseline chart audit (N = 7) (October 2009).

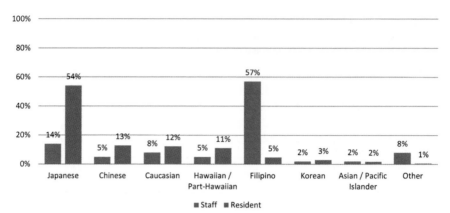

Fig. 4. Leahi Hospital ethnicity demographics resident and staff (July 2009).

IMPLEMENTATION STRATEGIES

The Iowa Model of Evidence-Based Practice to Promote Quality of Care[15] guided the process. The project team established a standardized, system-wide interdisciplinary approach to pain management to optimize multidisciplinary practice and resident outcomes.

The goals of the facility's evidence-based pain assessment and management program included (1) prompt assessment and diagnosis of pain; (2) use of appropriate pain scales for both cognitively intact and cognitively impaired residents; (3) pain treatment techniques based on standards of practice; (4) steps to monitor treatment effectiveness; (5) improvement of resident well-being by increasing comfort; (6) optimizing the resident's ability to perform activities of daily living and participate in activities; (7) monitoring for side effects of prevention/treatment related to the use of pain medications; and (8) monitoring and evaluating the effectiveness of the pain management care plan. Although the focus of the project was to improve pain assessment of cognitively impaired elderly, the Core Team also identified the need to address pain management in its entirety—screening, assessing, and monitoring.

The facility's direct care nursing staff (ie, RNs, LPNs, CNAs, and Patient Care Technicians) represented 86% of all clinical staff. Most of the nursing staff was foreign born and educated outside United States. The use of English as a second language has been problematic for some of these nursing staff members; a situation complicated by cultural differences in work expectations and performance. Therefore, education on new pain assessment practices needed to address the special needs of this group to increase the chances of successful implementation of the desired practice change. Educational materials for staff inservice training were created and/or modified to include content and examples using translation of key words into Ilocano and Tagalog for clarification and understanding (**Table 3**). Also included were familiar and culturally relevant clinical scenario case studies and demonstrations.

The didactic content was delivered via interactive lectures and demonstrations conducted by the Educational Director and members of the Core Team; case studies were used as the basis for group discussions, practical exercises, and small group work. Training was required and tailored to the clinical role of staff members, including overview of the revised pain assessment policy and management program, use of the PAINAD tool, and pain monitoring flowsheet forms relevant to the staff member's clinical role.

Under the leadership of all nurse managers, the practice change was implemented on all 5 resident care nursing units. Following training of staff, the PAINAD tool, comprehensive pain assessment form, and pain monitoring flowsheet were piloted housewide for 60 days with all licensed nursing staff (RNs and LPNs) who cared for residents who are cognitively impaired. The PAINAD tool was completed by the nursing staff and took approximately 3 minutes to complete.

As a result of the pilot, the team made necessary modifications to the EBP pain standard and instituted the change in practice by (1) revising the pain policy and procedure; (2) implementing the modification housewide by providing additional inservice education as appropriate to all clinical staff; (3) continuing to perform quarterly chart audits and on-the-spot review/evaluation with staff as necessary; and (4) providing

Table 3
Pain assessment in advance dementia (PAINAD) scale: Tagalog and Ilocano translation

Leahi Hospital

Pain Assessment in Advance Dementia (PAINAD) Scale -Tagalog Translation

	0	1	2	Score
Breathing Independent Of vocalization *Paghinga *Walang reklamo	Normal *Normal na Paghinga	Occasional labored Breathing, Short Period of Hyperventilation *Paminsan-minsan Nahirapang huminga *Malalim at madalang huminga	Noisy labored Long period of Hyperventilation Chyne-strokes Respirations *Maingay, Mahaba, mabilis ang paghinga. *Paghinga ay parang Naghihingalo.	
Negative Vocalization *Maraming reklamo	None *Walang reklamo	Occasional moan Or groan Low level speech With negative or Disapproving Quality *Paminsang-nimsang dumadaing. *Mahina ang boses	Reapeated troubled calling Out. Loud moaning or groaning. Crying *Paulit-ulit na tumatawag *Dumadaing na malakas *Umiiyak	
Facial Expression *Itsura ng Mukha	Smiling or Inexpressive * Nakangiti	Sad, Frightened, Frown *Matamlay o malungkot, natatakot o nakasimangot	Facial Grimacing *Nakasimangot	
Body Language *kilos ng katawan	Relaxed *Nakarelaks	Tense, Distressed, Pacing Fidgeting *Naninigas *Dimapakali	Rigid, Fists clenched Knees pulled up Pulling or pushing away Striking out *Naninigas at nakatikom Ang kamao. *Nakataas and tuhod o kaya hinihilang palayo o Nanunulak o manununtok	
Consolability *Suyuin	No Need to Console *Hindi kailangang suyuin	Distractred or reassured by voice Or touch *Wala sa sarili *Kailangang suyuin o haplosin	Unable to console- Distract or reassure *Hindi mapakiusapan	

(continued on next page)

Table 3
(continued)

Pain Assessment in Advance Dementia (PAINAD) Scale - Ilocano Translation

	0	1	2	Score
Breathing Independent of vocalization *Pinaganges *Awan reclamo	Normal *Kadawyan a pinaganges	Occasional labored Breathing. Short period of Hyperventilation *Sagpaminsan nga marigatan nga aganges, wenno nauneg ti pinaganges	Noisy labored Breathing. Long period of hyperventilation. Cheyne-strokes respirations. *Naringor, umanangsab ti anges na. *Marigatan nga aganges.	
Negative Vocalization *Adu ti reclamo	None *Awan ti nasakit	Occasional moan or groan. Low level speech with a negative or disapproving quality. *Sagpaminsan nga agongol. * Agtantanamitim	Repeated troubled calling out. Loud moaning or groaning. Crying * Pauli-ulit nga ag-tawtawag wenno agpukpukaw. *Napigsa nga agas-asug, wenno agsangsangit	
Facial Expression *Langa ti rupa	Smiling, or inex-pressive. *Umisisem *Nalawag ti rupa na	Sad, frightened, Frown * Naliday, mabuteng ti langana * Nakamisuot	Facial Grimacing * Nakamuregreg	
Body language *Gunay ti bagi	Relaxed * Natalna	Tense, Distressed Pacing, Fidgeting *Madimakatalna	Rigid, fists clenched, Knees pulled up, Pulling away or pushing away; Striking out *Agpatpatangken, nakagemgem ti ima na, ikukot na diay tumeng na no masagid wenno kumabil pay.	
Consolability *Ayayo	No need to console * Madi na masapul ti ayayo	Distracted or reassured by voice or touch *Masapul na ti ayayo wenno apros	Unable console, distract or reassure. *Madi dumngeg ti sarita wenno madi nga maayayo	

Data from Warden V, Hurley AC, Volicer L. Development and psychometric evaluation of the pain assessment in advanced dementia (PAINAD) scale. J Am Med Dir Assoc 2003;4(1):9–15. Translated to Ilocano by Myrna Galang, RN and Carlina Marquez, RN, for training purposes.

visual reminders and other resources for staff. To integrate the practice change permanently into nursing practice, the EBP standard and pain program/curriculum were incorporated in the nursing orientation and offered annually to the nursing staff thereafter, or as necessary.

EVALUATION

The final results of the authors' project included (1) chart audits (N = 23) to measure nursing staff's documentation compliance with new standards, (2) informal qualitative staff feedback on satisfaction with new tools, (3) factors that facilitated and/or hindered the implementation of the pain assessment, (4) evaluation of the nursing staff's competency using the PAINAD tool, and (5) modification of the standard based on the results.

As a result of the change in practice, significant improvement was noted in the nursing staff's comprehensive assessment of resident pain and documentation compliance (**Fig. 5**). Specifically, in monitoring for side effects of analgesics (60% improvement), nondrug interventions included in plan of care (33% improvement), pain care plan in place (9% improvement), pain scale tool used identified in care plan (51% improvement); and completed comprehensive pain assessment (71% improvement).

LESSONS LEARNED/RECOMMENDATIONS

Overall, staff education approaches proved to be the most important factor in the success of implementing this evidence-based nursing practice change. Translation of the PAINAD tool to Ilocano and Tagalog languages and customizing the education of nursing staff using clinical scenarios common to the cultural diversity of the residents and staff ethnicity improved their comprehension of pain-related behaviors in residents with cognitive deficits. Three of the nurse managers who participated in the education of staff also spoke Ilocano, Tagalog, and Visayan languages that were prevalent among the Filipino nursing staff. These managers taught at the training sessions, reinforced the use of the PAINAD tool on the units, and often translated concepts using the staff members' primary language to interpret standards as needed; this was especially important among CNAs who had primary roles as the direct caregivers of residents and served as first-line staff to recognize pain-related behavior and report such observations to the charge nurse on duty.

The use of the MASSPRO[14] guideline for an interdisciplinary approach to pain management was effective in ensuring all levels of disciplines involved in resident care at this facility provided input and participated in the project. This Interdisciplinary Committee consisted of the Medical Director; a Geriatric Psychiatrist; an Assistant Administrator; Department Heads of Rehabilitation, Social Services, Food Service, Recreation Therapy, Pharmacy, Quality Assurance, Education, as well as Nursing

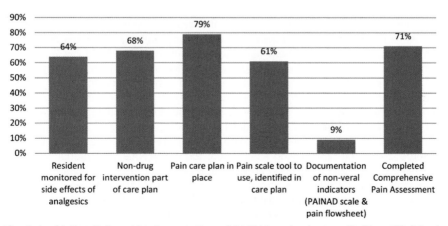

Fig. 5. Leahi Hospital post-implementation of PAINAD scale chart audit (N = 23) (March 2010).

Administration; Nurse Managers; and Coordinators. The involvement of this Interdisciplinary Committee in the project ensured important "buy-in" of the changes that were being made, even if the practice change of the project primarily targeted nursing assessment; this was most effective among the nonnursing clinical staff who also learned about the revised screening tools for pain assessment with cognitively impaired residents and incorporated changes into their respective disciplinary documentation in the medical record. This "buy-in" created a common housewide standard for pain identification and documentation, as well as a system-wide approach to pain management. The committee also provided a forum to discuss other related topics, such as effective analgesic pain management and care plan protocols to address complications of opioid use.

Although the use of the Interdisciplinary Committee was important, on-going meetings with this group were difficult to schedule, given the complex schedules of all the participants and their competing priorities. It was also acknowledged that some of the interests of the larger committee detracted from the main goal of the project, delaying decision making. It was decided to have the Interdisciplinary Committee serve as an advisory group that would meet as needed and would be kept informed of the project's progress.

The Iowa Model of Evidence-Based Practice to Promote Quality of Care[15] guided the project's process. One key aspect of the Iowa Model that was a challenge was the scope of the pilot. Although it may have been beneficial to pilot on a smaller scale such as one unit, staff and leadership wanted to pilot on all units for 60 days. All Nursing Unit Managers participated in the baseline data collection, research, and critique of research and practice and collectively determined the best EBP that was desired; all thus favored piloting the change on each of the 5 units of the facility. This meant a housewide pilot, which required education of all nursing staff including regularly assigned staff on units, float or relief staff. In retrospect, the Core Team realized the impact of implementing housewide. Piloting on a smaller scale may have provided an opportunity to assess barriers to the practice change, which may have assisted in refining implementation strategies.

Evaluation of the program included informal qualitative feedback from the nurses regarding factors that facilitated and/or hindered the implementation of EB pain assessment practices. Additionally, the medical record documentation system at this facility was largely noncomputerized, narrative, and often found to be incomplete and occasionally illegible.

Nursing staff members benefited from the practice change because the new assessment was reported to require less time, approximately 3 minutes compared with 10 minutes per assessment using the current tools (the Doloplus-2 and the Wong-Baker pain scales). They also gained knowledge about pain assessment by way of the educational intervention and changed their practice for better patient care. Residents benefited from decreased burden of time for assessments and, more importantly, increased accuracy of pain assessment resulting in appropriate and timely pain management interventions.

To sustain the practice, the team recommended to (1) continue to educate staff and reinforce use of the new/revised assessment forms (PAINAD, Comprehensive Pain Assessment, and pain monitoring flowsheet); (2) conduct monthly audits on appropriate use of the PAINAD assessment form (for residents with cognitive impairment/communication difficulties) and pain monitoring flowsheet (for all residents) with signs and symptoms of pain and who are on routine/PRN meds; (3) continue IDT review of Comprehensive Pain Assessment during resident's quarterly care conference if resident is coded for pain symptoms on MDS; (4) continue trending nursing compliance through monthly chart audits; and (5) report findings to the Hospital Quality Assurance and Assessment Committee.

SUMMARY

The purpose of this project was to identify best practices for pain identification in residents with cognitive impairment and institutionalize a standardized evidence-based pain assessment guide to optimize nursing practice and resident outcomes. The project was conducted in 2 phases: (1) Phase I analyzed data gained from chart reviews on current practices of pain assessment and (2) Phase II used the results of Phase I to develop, implement, and evaluate EBPs for nursing assessment of pain in cognitively impaired residents.

The key to pain management is recognizing that a resident is in pain. Pain assessments for residents in LTC facilities are often complicated by changes in memory, language skills, abstraction, and difficulties conceptualizing distress as pain. These complications can make assessment and intervention even more difficult. Hence, as CMS implemented changes in comprehensive pain assessment instructions in April 2009, the Nurse Managers identified a need to improve current assessment tools, continue staff education, and promote awareness of effectively assessing and documenting pain in residents with cognitive impairment. The former Doloplus-2 Pain Assessment Scale was difficult for nursing staff to understand and use in practice and required an excessive amount of time to complete; this further prompted the need to pursue this evidence-based project.

The success of this project was due to the implementation of EBPs including the following: (1) understanding the challenges to successfully evaluate and manage pain in patients with communication difficulties due to illness or language and cultural barriers, stoicism about pain, and cognitive impairment[8–10]; (2) recognizing that nurses are the key to effective pain management, however, may lack pain knowledge necessary to assess and manage their residents' pain effectively[5]; and (3) understanding that effective assessment and management of pain in cognitively impaired residents will result in improved outcomes and improved quality of life.

In addition, the harnessing of both interdisciplinary input and multicultural expertise led to a richer involvement of a diverse health care team that ultimately resulted in an institutional culture change in the assessment and management of pain.

REFERENCES

1. Department of Health & Human Services (DHHS) & Centers for Medicare & Medicaid Services (CMS). Revisions to Appendices P and PP. CMS Manual System. 2009. Available at: http://www.cms.gov/Regulations-and-Guidance/Guidance/Transmittals/downloads/R41SOMA.pdf. Accessed July 22, 2013.
2. Department of Health & Human Services (DHHS) & Centers for Medicare & Medicaid Services (CMS). Minimum Data Set 3.0 Public Reports. 2012. Available at: http://www.cms.gov/Research-Statistics-Data-and-Systems/Computer-Data-and-%09Systems/Minimum-Data-Set-3-0-Public-Reports/index.html. Accessed July 22, 2013.
3. Mauk K, Hanson P. Management of common illnesses, diseases, and health conditions. In: Mauk K, editor. Gerontological nursing: competencies for care. Sudbury (MA): Jones and Bartlett; 2009. p. 382–453.
4. Kaufman M. When it hurts: caring for the older adult in pain. 2006. Available at: http://www.nursing.upenn.edu/cisa/geroTIPS/tlcltc/Documents/9_pain-07.pdf. Accessed July 22, 2013.

5. Textor LH, Porock D. The pain management knowledge of nurses practicing in a rural midwest retirement community. J Nurses Staff Dev 2006;22:307–12.
6. Lefebre-Chapiro L, Doloplus group. The Doloplus 2 scale-evaluating pain in the elderly. Eur J of Palliative Care 2001;8:191–4.
7. Wong DL, Hockenberry-Eaton M, Wilson D, et al. Wong–Baker faces. Wong's essentials of pediatric nursing. 6th edition. St Louis (MO): Mosby, Inc; 2001. p. 1301.
8. Cohen-Mansfield J. Pain assessment in noncommunicative elderly persons – PAINE. Clin J Pain 2006;22(6):569–75.
9. Jones K, Fink R, Clark L, et al. Nursing home resident barriers to effective pain management: why nursing home residents may not seek pain medication. J Am Med Dir Assoc 2005;6(1):10–7.
10. Yong HH, Gibson SJ, Horne DJ, et al. Development of a pain attitudes questionnaire to assess stoicism and cautiousness for possible age differences. J Gerontol B Psychol Sci Soc Sci 2001;56:279–84.
11. Cluzeau FA, Burgers JS, Brouwers M, et al. Development and validation of an international appraisal instrument for assessing the quality of clinical practice guidelines: the AGREE project. Qual Saf Health Care 2003;12(1):18–23.
12. Warden V, Hurley AC, Volicer L. Development and psychometric evaluation of the pain assessment in advanced dementia (PAINAD) scale. J Am Med Dir Assoc 2003;4(1):9–15. Available at: http://www.healthcare.uiowa.edu/igec/tools/pain/PAINAD.pdf. Accessed October 29, 2013.
13. Herr K, Bjoro K, Decker S. Tools for assessment of pain in nonverbal older adults with dementia: a state-of-the-science review. J Pain Symptom Manage 2006; 31(2):170–92.
14. Medicare Quality Improvement Organization for Massachusetts. A systems approach to quality improvement in long-term care: Pain Management. 2006. Available at: http://ltctoolkit.rnao.ca/sites/ltc/files/resources/pain/NHPainManual_Nov2006e.pdf. Accessed October 29, 2013.
15. Titler M, Kleiber C, Rakel B, et al. A conceptual model for growing evidence-based practice. Nurs Adm Q 2007;31(2):162–70.

Pulmonary Management of the Acute Cervical Spinal Cord Injured Patients

Katherine G. Johnson, MS, RN, APRN, CCRN, CNRN, CNS-BC*,
Leilani Jean B. Hill, BSN, RN

KEYWORDS

- Pulmonary • Cervical spine • Acute injury • Respiration

KEY POINTS

- Respiratory complications are a common cause of morbidity and mortality in patients with acute cervical spinal cord injury and treatments must be initiated immediately.
- The longer it takes for a patient to receive pulmonary treatments and mobility activities, the higher the morbidity and mortality and the longer the length of stay.
- Disrupted pulmonary mechanics and respiratory complications are frequent and are influenced by the level of injury.

INTRODUCTION
Background

A traumatic spinal cord injury (SCI) is a catastrophic event associated with physiologic disruptions to the motor, sensory, cardiovascular, and respiratory systems. Regardless of the level of injury, pulmonary mechanics of the chest muscles, upper abdomen, and diaphragm are frequently altered.[1] An acute cervical SCI (acSCI) severely compromises respiratory function because of paralysis and impairment of the respiratory muscles.[2] More than half (54%) of all SCIs occur at the cervical level.[3] Atelectasis, pneumonia, and ventilatory failure affect as many as 84% of patients with the higher C1 to C4 SCIs.[4–6] Patients with lower cervical and thoracic lesions also have compromised respiratory function requiring diligent clinical assessments.[4]

Altered pulmonary function and complications are the leading cause of morbidity in patients with acute SCIs.[6–10] According to Winslow and colleagues,[11] the number of

Funding: This project was partially funded by the Agency for Healthcare Research & Quality, 5R13HS017892; Hawaii State Center for Nursing; and Queen Emma Nursing Institute, The Queen's Medical Center, Honolulu, HI.
The Queen's Medical Center, 1301 Punchbowl Street, Honolulu, HI 96813, USA
* Corresponding author.
E-mail address: KJohnson@queens.org

respiratory complications experienced during the initial acute-care hospitalization for SCI is a more important determinant of length of stay (LOS) and hospital costs than level of injury. The need for mechanical ventilation, development of pneumonia, need for surgery, and use of a tracheostomy account for 60% of hospital costs of patients with an SCI.[8]

Disrupted pulmonary mechanics and respiratory complications are frequent and are influenced by the level of injury. Therefore, identifying interventions that can minimize the need for mechanical ventilation and prevent respiratory complications are of great importance and are critical to begin immediately after injury.[6,8,10]

Triggers

The Iowa model of evidence-based practice was the framework used to guide this project.[12] The initial phase of the model focuses on problem and knowledge triggers and alignment with organizational priorities. Triggers identified by the primary project coordinators (nurse manager, change champion, and opinion leader) focused on improving collaborative care provided to patients with acSCI, predominantly in the area of pulmonary management. The coordinators thought that an improvement in the care delivery process had the potential to enhance patient outcomes, facilitate multidisciplinary collaboration, and reduce intensive care unit (ICU) LOS. These problem triggers are all areas that the organization considered as priorities.

A baseline chart review (April 2008 to June 2009) of 19 patients with acSCI in an 8-bed neuroscience ICU (NSICU), at a 500-bed level II trauma center, revealed an ICU LOS between 5 and 33 days (**Table 1**). Therefore, this article describes the process of developing an evidence-based guideline to reduce pulmonary complications and ICU LOS in the acute phase for cervical spinal cord injured patients.

Forming a Team

The next phase of the Iowa model focuses on selection of team members. A multidisciplinary team was strategically chosen from a variety of stakeholders representing

Table 1 SCI patient data		
	Baseline (n = 19) April 2008–June 2009	After Guidelines (n = 6) July 2011–Sept 2011
% Male	74	100
Average age (y)	37.4	36
Age ≤ 20 y (%)	21	50
Age ≥ 75 y (%)	5	17
Time to OR (Mean)		
≤24 h (%)	67 (n = 13)	100 (n = 4)
≤48 h (%)	11 (n = 2)	—
>48 h (%)	17 (n = 3)	—
Endotracheal Intubation (%)	53	100
Tracheostomy (%)	32	100
Tracheostomy day (mean)	8	8
Documentation of OOB (%)	74	100
First day OOB (mean)	11	7
ICU LOS, nontransferred survivors ICU mortality (%)	13 (5–33) (n = 15) 0	21 (17–27) (n = 4) 33

Abbreviations: OOB, out of bed; OR, operating room.

nursing, respiratory care, physical therapy, occupational therapy, and medicine (**Box 1**). Monthly meetings were held for 2 hours for a year to critique and synthesize literature and develop the practice guideline.

EVIDENCE FOR PRACTICE IMPROVEMENT
Literature Review

PubMed and CINAHL (Cumulative Index to Nursing and Allied Health Literature) databases were used to search terms related to respiratory or pulmonary complications in patients with acSCI. Thirty articles dated between 2000 and 2009 consisting of published guidelines, meta-analyses, randomized and nonrandomized controlled trials, retrospective chart reviews, and review articles were critiqued by the team (**Table 2**) using Mosby levels of evidence.[13] After the initial review, an additional 6 articles were reviewed and critiqued for consideration for inclusion in future guideline revisions.

Literature Critique

Invasive versus noninvasive ventilation
Noninvasive ventilation is a potential alternative to traditional ventilation following an SCI for select patients.[7,8,10,14] Noninvasive techniques preserve the patient's natural pulmonary defense mechanisms, averting bacterial colonization and inflammation associated with intubation and tracheotomies.[8] Wong and colleagues[6] suggest that patients with incomplete motor injuries below C5 may be candidates for noninvasive techniques such as bi-level positive airway pressure (Bi-PAP) ventilation, positive end-expiratory pressure (PEEP) therapy, vibratory therapy, or lung expansion therapies such as deep breathing and coughing. Patients prefer noninvasive ventilation for comfort, the ability to retain their swallow function, and the ability to communicate.[9]

In patients with injuries that allow spontaneous breathing, safety measures such as close monitoring for impending respiratory failure and measuring of respiratory mechanics such as vital capacity are recommended.[4] Patients with signs of respiratory

---

Box 1
Multidisciplinary team members

Change champion

Opinion leaders

Evidence-based practice resources

NSICU staff nurses

NSICU nurse manager

Clinical nurse specialist

Neuroscience intensivist (ad hoc)

Neurologic surgeon (ad hoc)

Respiratory therapists

Respiratory therapist clinical educator

Respiratory therapist manager

Physical therapist

Nursing student

Table 2	
Levels of evidence	
Number of Articles (n = 30)	**Evidence Level**
1	Meta-analysis (level I)
3	Randomized control trial, well designed (level II)
1	Controlled trial, no randomization (level III)
3	Case controlled or cohort studies (level IV)
0	Correlational study (level V)
12	Single descriptive or qualitative study (level VI)
0	Authority opinion or expert committee report (level VII)
7	Review articles (other) or performance improvement
3	Guideline

Adapted from Melnyk B. A focus on adult acute and critical care. Worldviews Evid Based Nurs 2004;1(3):195; with permission.

failure such as tachypnea, hypoxia, diminished cough, and a vital capacity less than 15 mL/kg of body weight should be considered for intubation.[1,8]

A retrospective chart review performed by Velmahos and colleagues[15] on 68 patients with SCI found risk factors that predicted a patient's likelihood of the need for endotracheal intubation. The 3 independent risk factors were an injury severity score greater than 16, a cervical cord injury higher than C5, and complete quadriplegia. The combination of a cervical spinal injury at a level higher than C5 and complete quadriplegia resulted in intubation of 95% of patients.

The decision to support a patient with SCI with either invasive or noninvasive ventilator interventions is defined by the level and extent of the injury. Regardless, patients need to be supported through their initial acute phase of recovery, frequently monitored, and cared for by providers knowledgeable in their unique needs.

Prevention of atelectasis and pneumonia

Management of atelectasis is an important component of early respiratory care. Atelectasis develops secondary to an impaired expansion of the lung caused by weak respiratory muscles, abdominal contents, retained bronchial secretions, and a weak cough. Atelectasis may worsen during the patients' first few days as respiratory muscles fatigue, secretions accumulate, and lung compliance decreases.[6] Suggested interventions to reexpand affected lung tissues are listed in **Table 3**.

In addition, a comprehensive protocol to prevent ventilator-associated pneumonia is highly encouraged.[12] Interventions such as deep vein thrombosis prophylaxis, gastrointestinal prophylaxis, use of an endotracheal tube with subglottic secretion drainage, and oral care with chlorhexidine gluconate solution may help to prevent pneumonia.

Secretion management

Hypersecretion of bronchial mucus occurs within 1 hour in greater than 40% of individuals with acSCI and quadriplegia.[8] Increased secretions with an ineffective cough and bronchospasm leads to mucous plugs, commonly seen during the first 5 days. Secretions are abnormal in both amount and chemical content, but this abnormality tends to return to normal over the subsequent months.[8] Suggested secretion management interventions are listed in **Table 4**.

Tracheal suctioning is often insufficient for secretion mobilization. Retained secretions caused by expiratory muscle weakness are treated with manually assisted

Table 3
Lung expansion interventions

Lung Expansion Interventions	Lung Expansion Interventions (with Endotracheal Tubes)
Deep breathing and voluntary coughing	Intermittent positive pressure breathing
Assisted coughing techniques (quad cough)	Sigh breaths
Glossopharyngeal breathing	Mechanical insufflation-exsufflation treatment
Incentive spirometry	Tidal volumes >20 mL/kg
Chest physical therapy	Oral gastric tubes for decompression
Continuous positive airway pressure	Fiber optic bronchoscopy with bronchoalveolar
Bi-PAP	lavage
Supine or Trendelenburg positions	EzPAP positive airway pressure system
Use of abdominal binders	Acapella

Data from Refs.[1,6,8,11]

maneuvers such as assisted coughing or mechanical insufflation-exsufflation. The mechanical insufflation-exsufflation device produces a cough flow comparable with a normal cough and that can be administered via tracheotomy or mouth, and that is well tolerated by patients[1]; patients prefer this device to suctioning.[16]

Surgery

Surgery after a traumatic SCI typically involves stabilization and decompression of neural tissue; however, controversy still exists regarding the potential neurologic benefits and timing.[17–19] There is some evidence that early surgery for decompression may improve neurologic recovery and that it can be performed safely within less than 24 hours after acute SCI.[17] According to McKinley and colleagues,[19] surgery within 72 hours is associated with earlier transition to rehabilitation and decreased overall hospital LOS.

A meta-analysis of 1687 patients showed that 90% of patients with incomplete SCI improved neurologically after early decompression.[18] However, when all other clinical factors were considered, investigators recommended that early surgery be considered as a practice option only. Late surgeries were noted to be related to significant increases in acute-care requirements and total LOS, higher hospital charges, and a higher incidence of pneumonia and atelectasis.[19] This finding is potentially caused by activity restrictions that are frequently placed on a patient before surgical fixation.

Table 4
Secretion management interventions

Secretion Management Interventions	Secretion Management Interventions for Patients with Endotracheal Tubes
Assisted coughing/quad cough	High-frequency percussive ventilation[6]
Incentive spirometry	T-piece trials/tubing compensation
Mechanical insufflator/exsufflator	Pressure support
EzPAP positive airway pressure system	Pulmonary toilet
Glossopharyngeal breathing	Warm moist air
Chest physiotherapy-vest treatment	Bronchodilators/mucolytics,
Continuous positive airway pressure/Bi-PAP	PEEP
Trendelenburg/supine position	
Rotating beds	
Postural drainage	
Bronchoscopy	

Data from Refs.[1,6,9–11,16]

The timing of surgical treatment of a patient with acute SCI remains in debate. Early surgery decreases pulmonary complications, shortens hospitalizations, and decreases overall hospital charges, but there is no agreement on optimal timing or neurologic benefit.[17] Initiation of early discussion with the health care team regarding the timing of surgery might prove beneficial.

Tracheostomy

Patients who are expected to have prolonged or permanent respiratory failure after an SCI undergo tracheotomies. A tracheotomy is more comfortable for the patient, easier to suction, easier to perform pulmonary hygiene, and easier to wean from the ventilator because of less dead space and reduced airway resistance.[5,8] It also decreases the need for sedation, increases mobility, improves patient communication, and decreases pulmonary complications, all directly affecting the overall hospital and ICU LOS.[5]

Approximately 10% of patients who remain ventilator dependent for more than 24 hours in the ICU eventually require a tracheotomy.[20] A retrospective chart review by Leelapattana and colleagues[5] of 66 patients in a Canadian hospital sought to identify patients who were likely to need prolonged mechanical ventilation and would benefit from an early tracheotomy. Their group recommended early tracheotomy if the patient's injury severity score (ISS) is greater than 32, the patient has a complete SCI, and acute lung injury (Pao_2/fraction of inspired oxygen ratio <300) is present on day 3. They showed that the number of days in the hospital increased by 2.3 days for every additional day from injury to tracheotomy.

A retrospective chart review of 275 adult survivors of acSCI found that 76% of patients with complete SCI impairments (American Spinal Injury Association [ASIA] A, absence of sensory or motor function) underwent a tracheotomy.[21] The median time from anterior spine fixation and tracheotomy was 7 days and 71% of the tracheotomies were performed via a percutaneous procedure. None of the patients developed a wound infection. These investigators support the safety of a percutaneous tracheotomy 6 to 10 days after an anterior cervical fusion.

A second retrospective chart review of 20 patients who underwent an anterior cervical fusion (ACF) and received a postfixation tracheotomy was described.[22] This review revealed that half of the patients had postfixation tracheotomy at a mean of 6.9 days (range 0–17 days) after their ACF and no wound or implant infection occurred in any patient. Another retrospective chart review of 319 patients with SCI in a Japanese hospital revealed that risk factors predictive of the need for a tracheotomy included patients older than 69 years, severe ASIA impairment scale,[23] low forced vital capacity ($\leq$500 mL), and low percent vital capacity (<16.3%).[24]

Tracheotomy placement before day 7 offers the advantages of shortened mechanical ventilation, reduced ICU LOS, and lower rates of tracheal intubation complications.[7,25]

Activity/Mobility

Inactivity in patients with SCI has been associated with secondary health problems such as pressure ulcers, depression, and chronic pain.[26] The Consortium for Spinal Cord Medicine[27] and a review article by Ginis and colleagues[26] reported that early physical activity may prevent secondary disease and complications, but limited data are provided to support this hypothesis. Therefore, the health care team should establish when it would be appropriate and safe for a patient with SCI to start rehabilitation therapy.

Multiple health care disciplines coordinate care to promote early mobility. Development of upright positioning protocols, orthostatic hypotension management, pressure relief strategies, and patient/family education are shared among the members of the health care team. Nurses apply lower limb compression devices and abdominal binders, ensure hemodynamic stability with upright positioning, and provide passive range of motion assistance. Physical therapy treatments include range of motion and strengthening exercises, proper seating and positioning, dangling at the bedside, and edema management. Occupational therapy treatment includes range of motion, strengthening, and stretching exercises; upper and lower extremity splint fabrication; position and seating; retraining for activities of daily living; and mobilization that includes bed mobility and transfer training.

Speech and swallow

Speech and language disorder treatments include functional and/or augmentative communication, assessment of swallowing, as well as patient and/or family education. Swallowing dysfunction, or dysphagia, following an SCI is an under-recognized complication that can occur in up to 40% of quadriplegic patients.[8] The most common complications of dysphagia are airway obstruction, chemical pneumonitis, and pneumonia.[28] A prospective study by Chaw and colleagues[28] found that the presence of a tracheotomy, ventilator use, and the presence of a nasogastric tube were all predictors of dysphagia in patients with SCI. An evaluation of swallowing function should be done before oral feeding in any patient with an acSCI, halo fixation, cervical spine surgery, prolonged intubation, or tracheotomy.[27,28]

Practice Recommendations

The evidence suggests that all spinal cord injured patients, especially those involving cervical injuries, benefit from immediate respiratory interventions. Multiple medical, respiratory, nursing, and rehabilitation treatments were found to be effective methods to minimize pulmonary complications and reduce LOS. Treatments such as the use of noninvasive ventilation, lung inflation, secretion management, timing of tracheotomy (early; within 7 days), early surgical repair, and activity/mobility measures were all interventions that influence the rate of complications and overall LOS.

Based on the evidence, the team formulated interventions to minimize pulmonary complications, such as (1) secretion management, (2) prevention of atelectasis, (3) consideration for noninvasive ventilation, (3) encouraging timely surgery, (4) supporting timely tracheotomy placement, and (5) facilitating activity/mobility. These interventions were chosen by the team to incorporate into the evidence-based guideline. Future guideline revisions will consider including dysphagia management in the bedside checklist and ventilator weaning protocols designed for patients with SCI.

IMPLEMENTATION STRATEGIES
Piloting and Instituting the Practice Change

Baseline data and outcomes

Outcomes were selected based on the evidence and triggers. The objective of this project was to develop and disseminate an evidence-based guideline to support collaborative care of acute spinal cord injured patients. Recommended medical, nursing, respiratory, and rehabilitation interventions were incorporated in order to reduce the ICU LOS. Data were collected for the use of invasive ventilation, time to tracheotomy, timing of surgical stabilization, as well as out of bed (OOB) activities to determine effectiveness of the practice change.

Guideline development

The team spent 10 months developing the guideline, "Pulmonary Management of the Acute Cervical Spinal Cord Injured Patient–Evidence Based Practice Guideline." The guideline consisted of a review of the literature, a decision algorithm (**Fig. 1**), and a bedside checklist (**Fig. 2**) incorporating a synthesis of the available evidence. Current respiratory therapy protocols for secretion management and lung inflation were revised to support the needs of patients with SCI and were included in the guideline. Final support was gained from the various stakeholders, such as the unit-based intensivists; neurosurgery and pulmonary consultants; and nursing, rehabilitation, and respiratory therapy staff members.

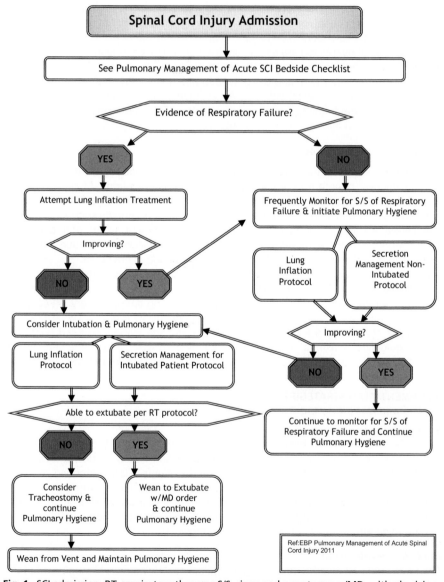

Fig. 1. SCI admission. RT, respiratory therapy; S/S, signs and symptoms; w/MD, with physician.

Admission	Day 1	Day 2	Day 3	Day 4	Day 5	Day 6	Day 7	APPENDIX
Lung Inflation Protocol								A. Spinal Cord Injury Admission Algorithm
Secretion Management Protocol per guideline								B. Lung Inflation SCI Protocol
ABG: (PRN)								C. Secretion Management SCI Protocol
NIF/VC:								D. Secretion Management (Intubated) SCI Protocol
IS: ___ L								E. S/S of Respiratory Fatigue
Chest x-ray: (PRN)								F. Types of Respiratory Protocols & Explanation
SCD:								G. Quad Cough Technique
Turn q2h (if not contraindicated)								H. Applying an Abdominal Binder
Abd binder use:								I. Applying Ted Hose
Quad Cough (if not contraindicated)								J. Rehabilitation Services (OT, PT, ST) Considerations
Ted Hose Use								
Operative Day?								NOTE – For many patients with Neuromuscular disorders or Spinal Cord
Trach Day?								Injuries (SCI), aggressive respiratory therapy may be required until they are discharged
Activity/OOB order?								home or to a Rehab Center. Other adjunct therapies may also be required such as
Thromboembolic Therapy?								Quad coughing maneuvers, the use of abdominal binders and other devices to
Pneumococcal Vaccination?								assist with airway clearance.

Fig. 2. Bedside checklist. ABG, arterial blood gas; NIF/VC, negative inspiratory force and vital capacity; OT, occupational therapist; PRN, as needed; PT, physical therapist; ST, speech therapist.

Guideline implementation
Education and marketing The pilot plan was to disseminate and implement the guideline in the NSICU. Dissemination and communication of the newly developed guideline was done through educational in-services, daily unit-based huddles, and hospital-wide nursing grand rounds. Educational in-services were done via unit-based competency fairs and multiple scheduled in-services for the nursing staff and respiratory therapists held twice a week, 4 times a day for 2 weeks. An in-service for the rehabilitation department was held during a staff meeting.

Resource binders containing items such as lung inflation and secretion management protocols, signs and symptoms of respiratory fatigue, and assisted coughing (quad cough) techniques were created for easy access on the nursing units. The team recommended that the checklist be initiated on admission and would be used to guide the staff coordinating daily treatments. These completed checklists were used to monitor compliance.

EVALUATION
Monitor and Analyze Structures

Outcomes
The pilot project was initially intended for patients admitted to the NSICU only. However, because of bed capacity issues, patients with acSCI were transferred to other ICU beds in the medical and surgical ICUs after their initial stabilization, which required additional in-servicing to the adjacent ICU units and created additional barriers to guideline compliance.

Evaluation was conducted via a checklist and chart review only for patients who remained in the NSICU. The baseline data (n = 19) and 3-month pilot data (n = 6) are displayed in **Table 1**. Two-thirds of the baseline patients received surgical stabilization within 24 hours; more than half required invasive intubation and one-third required a tracheotomy. For this group, the first day OOB was day 11 and OOB activities were documented for only 74% of patients. Mortality was 0% for this group and their ICU LOS was 13 days.

In the postguideline pilot group, 100% of the patients went to the operating room within 24 hours. Invasive intubation and a subsequent tracheotomy was required by 100% of the pilot group; this differs from an article published by Harrop and colleagues.[20] Their article reports a nationwide Swiss survey in which only 10% of patients who remained ventilator dependent for longer than 24 hours required a tracheostomy.[20] The mean day of tracheotomy was unchanged at 8 days for both groups. Documentation of OOB activities improved to 100% and occurred 4 days earlier than for the baseline group. Chart reviews revealed earlier use of sequential compression devices, antiembolic stockings, and abdominal binders.

The average ICU LOS in this small pilot group increased by 8 days, but the range of ICU stay was 17 to 27 days, or 6 days less than the baseline data (5–33 days). These differences in LOS were caused by clinical reasons related to ventilation/tracheotomy, as well as financial and community resources.

A postimplementation survey was sent out to staff nurses, respiratory therapists, rehabilitation services staff, Doctors of Medicine, and Advanced Practice Registered Nurses. Results indicated that most were aware of the guideline but only half of the subjects surveyed (n = 19) used the guideline. Reasons for the lack of use were related to accessibility. Thirty-two percent of the surveyed staff members were unaware of the guideline.

In summary, implementation of the guideline showed varying results. The postguideline patients were more severely injured, resulting in intubation and subsequent tracheostomy rather than noninvasive ventilator support. ICU LOS increased by 8 days, also reflecting a patient population that required intubation and tracheotomies. Also, discharge from the ICU was delayed because of financial/insurance and community support, nonclinical reasons that were not affected by the new guideline. As hoped, the first day OOB decreased, showing that patients could and were getting out of bed earlier; documentation reflecting more mobility interventions.

Dysphagia and its associated complications were not initially addressed by the guideline. However, after a more recent literature review, early evaluation and interventions to address dysphagia and aspiration precautions will be added to the next update. Ventilator-free protocols have been shown to benefit patients who are eligible for weaning[10] and future revisions of this guideline will also consider these types of weaning protocols.

LESSONS LEARNED
Instituting the Practice Change

Sustaining practice changes requires multiple strategies. Educational in-services or interactive educational sessions need to be scheduled on a regular basis to update current as well as newly hired staff members. Providing scheduled education also allows for administrative support and staff planning. Infrequent patient admissions necessitated reeducation and staff follow-up for each patient, a role our team did not clearly define. Providing infrastructure such as computer-based access to the guideline and its contents may have enhanced compliance, especially for the patients being cared for in the non-NSICU areas. Admission orders sets that reference the guideline may also be helpful for this infrequently admitted patient population.

Stakeholder input and multidisciplinary collaboration were necessary for the success of guideline development, particularly for a topic that is heavily influenced by other disciplines. Guideline adherence was less than ideal for the ICUs that did not normally care for patients with acSCI. The dissemination plan chosen was focused on educational in-services and this strategy would likely have been more effective if the initially chosen ICU was the only one to which patients were admitted. However, when patients were admitted to adjacent ICUs, compliance with the guideline decreased. Future recommendations should advocate for multiple strategies to strengthen the dissemination and communication of the practice change, which might have been facilitated with the assistance of the shared governance unit councils.

A recommendation would be for a dedicated team member to address the guideline for each new admission, regardless of the admitting ICU. At our facility, the trauma service initially evaluates patients with acSCI. Therefore, it would be ideal for all members of the trauma inpatient service to be educated about the guideline. Other recommendations would be to increase accessibility by including the guideline on a computer network[29] and to create order sets that make it easy for attending physicians and residents to order treatments in accordance with the guideline.

SUMMARY

Respiratory complications are a common cause of morbidity and mortality in patients with acSCI and treatments must be initiated immediately. This article describes the process of developing an evidence-based practice guideline to reduce pulmonary complications and ultimately LOS in patients with acSCI. The longer it takes for patients to receive pulmonary treatments and mobility activities, the higher the morbidity and mortality and the longer the LOS.

The Iowa model guided the practice change in our facility to promote the care of patients with acSCI in a more organized, evidence-based, and expeditious manner. All staff involved were asked on a postimplementation survey whether they thought that the care of patients with SCI had changed since the SCI evidence based practice (EBP) project was implemented. Some comments indicated that more aggressive treatments were being done earlier to improve patient outcomes and decrease LOS in ICUs, that prophylactic care does not hurt patients, and that patients seem to be getting OOB more.

Using the Iowa model to promote a practice change that is evidence-based has been a challenging, but rewarding, experience. Our statewide EBP workshop and internship program provided the necessary skill development, guidance, support, and especially encouragement throughout the project. Work continues because the change still needs to be hardwired on the nursing units. Also, as evidence becomes available, work is needed to continue to update the guideline and the staff to further promote and facilitate the evidence-based care for patients with SCIs.

Evidence-based practice changes begin with education and have the potential to transform the clinical setting and positively affect patient outcomes. Important elements to facilitate the EBP process include time, organizational and manager support, skills and education, and access to information.[29] We were fortunate that our Magnet designation supported the related research and evidence-based initiatives that are characteristic of excellence in nursing services.

ACKNOWLEDGMENTS

The authors would like to acknowledge Chris Aguillon, RT; Rachel Ariola, RN; Deborah Bransford, RN; Diane Brenessel, RT; Cherylee Chang, MD; Daniel Donovan, MD; Ron Govina, RN; Kawehi Kauhola, RN; Stephen Kaya, RT; Renee Latimer, RN; Danny Le, RT; Debra Mark, RN; John Mauliola, PT; and Jenelle Palisca, RN for their support of this project.

REFERENCES

1. Consortium for Spinal Cord Medicine. Respiratory management following spinal cord injury: a clinical practice guideline. Washington, DC: Paralyzed Veterans of America; 2008.
2. Zimmer MB, Nantwi K, Goshgarian HG. Effect of spinal cord injury on the respiratory system: basic research and current clinical treatment options. J Spinal Cord Med 2007;30:319–30.
3. National Spinal Cord Injury Statistical Center. Spinal cord injury facts and figures at a glance, February 2013. NSCISC National Spinal Cord Injury Statistical Center; 2013. Available at: https://www.nscisc.uab.edu/PublicDocuments/fact_figures_docs/Facts%202013.pdf. Accessed November 23, 2013.
4. Hassid VJ, Schinco MA, Tepas JJ, et al. Definitive establishment of airway control is critical for optimal outcome in lower cervical spinal cord injury. J Trauma 2008; 65:1328–32.
5. Leelapattana P, Fleming JC, Gurr KR, et al. Predicting the need for tracheostomy in patients with cervical spinal cord injury. J Trauma Acute Care Surg 2012;73: 880–4.
6. Wong SL, Shem K, Crew J. Specialized respiratory management for acute cervical spinal cord injury: a retrospective analysis. Top Spinal Cord Inj Rehabil 2012; 18:283–90.
7. Ball PA. Critical care management of the patient with acute spinal cord injury. Spine 2001;26:S27–30.
8. Berlly M, Shem K. Respiratory management during the first five days after spinal cord injury. J Spinal Cord Med 2007;30:309–18.
9. Brown R, DiMarco AF, Hoit JD, et al. Respiratory dysfunction and management in spinal cord injury. Respir Care 2006;51:853–69.
10. Sheel A, Reid W, Townson A, et al. Respiratory management following spinal cord injury. In: Eng J, Teasell R, Miller W, et al, editors. Spinal cord injury rehabilitation evidence. Version 2. Vancouver (Canada): Spinal Cord Injury Rehabilitation Evidence [Project]; 2008. p. 8.1–8.40.
11. Winslow C, Bode RK, Felton D, et al. Impact of respiratory complications on length of stay and hospital costs in acute cervical spine injury. Chest 2002;121: 1548–54.
12. Titler MG, Kleiber C, Steelman VJ, et al. The Iowa model of evidence-based practice to promote quality care. Crit Care Nurs Clin North Am 2001;13: 497–509.
13. Melnyk BM. A focus on adult acute and critical care. Worldviews Evid Based Nurs 2004;1(3):194–7.
14. Bach JR, Hunt D, Horton JA 3rd. Traumatic tetraplegia: noninvasive respiratory management in the acute setting. Am J Phys Med Rehabil 2002;81:792–7.
15. Velmahos GC, Toutouzas K, Chan L, et al. Intubation after cervical spinal cord injury: to be done selectively or routinely? Am Surg 2003;69:891–4.

16. Schmitt JK, Stiens S, Trincher R, et al. Survey of use of the insufflator-exsufflator in patients with spinal cord injury. J Spinal Cord Med 2007;30:127–30.

17. Fehlings MG, Perrin RG. The timing of surgical intervention in the treatment of spinal cord injury: a systematic review of recent clinical evidence. Spine (Phila Pa 1976) 2006;31(Suppl 11):S28–35.

18. La Rosa G, Conti A, Cardali S, et al. Does early decompression improve neurological outcome of spinal cord injured patients? Appraisal of the literature using a meta-analytical approach. Spinal Cord 2004;42:503–12. Meta-analysis.

19. McKinley W, Meade MA, Kirshblum S, et al. Outcomes of early surgical management versus late or no surgical intervention after acute spinal cord injury. Arch Phys Med Rehabil 2004;85:1818–25.

20. Harrop J, Sharan A, Scheid E, et al. Tracheostomy placement in patients with complete cervical spinal cord injuries: American Spinal Cord Injury Association Grade A. J Neurosurg 2004;100(1 Suppl Spine):20–3.

21. O'Keeffe T, Goldman R, Mayberry JC, et al. Tracheostomy after anterior cervical spine fixation. J Trauma 2004;57:855–60.

22. Babu R, Owens TR, Thomas S, et al. Timing of tracheostomy after anterior cervical spine fixation. J Trauma Acute Care Surg 2013;74:961–6.

23. Ditunno JF Jr, Young W, Donovan WH, et al. The international standards booklet for neurological and functional classification of spinal cord injury. Paraplegia 1994;32:70–80.

24. Yugue I, Okada S, Ueta T, et al. Analysis of the risk factors for tracheostomy in traumatic cervical spinal cord injury. Spine (Phila Pa 1976) 2012;37:E1633–8.

25. Romero J, Vari A, Gambarrutta C, et al. Tracheostomy timing in traumatic spinal cord injury. Eur Spine J 2009;18:1452–7.

26. Martin Ginis KA, Latimer AE, Buchholz AC, et al. Establishing evidence-based physical activity guidelines: methods for the Study of Health and Activity in People with Spinal Cord Injury (SHAPE SCI). Spinal Cord 2008;46:216–21.

27. Consortium for Spinal Cord Medicine. Early acute management in adults with spinal cord injury: a clinical practice guideline for health professionals. Washington, DC: Paralyzed Veterans of America; 2005.

28. Chaw E, Shem K, Castillo K, et al. Dysphagia and associated respiratory considerations in cervical spinal cord injury. Top Spinal Cord Inj Rehabil 2012;18:291–9.

29. Melnyk BM, Fineout-Overholt E, Gallagher-Ford L, et al. The state of evidence-based practice in US nurses: critical implications for nurse leaders and educators. J Nurs Adm 2012;42:410–7.

Reducing Restraint Use in a Trauma Center Emergency Room

Rebecca Cole, RN, BS

KEYWORDS

- Restraints • Seclusion • Managing agitation • Emergency • Behavioral health
- Restraint reduction

KEY POINTS

- The use of seclusion and restraints has historically been described as a safe way to calm an agitated or violent patient in behavioral health care.
- Evidence supports reducing the use of restraints and seclusion because these episodes can result in psychological harm or physical injury to patients and staff.
- The culture in the Emergency Department has changed from reflexively applying restraints or using seclusion with an agitated patient to using noncoercive de-escalation techniques and attempting to develop a therapeutic relationship with the patient.

INTRODUCTION

The use of seclusion and restraints has historically been described as a safe way to calm an agitated or violent patient in behavioral health care. Recent evidence suggests that the use of seclusion and restraints can cause both psychological and physical injury to the patient and staff.[1] Deaths have been reported in the literature as a result of restraints or use of seclusion.[2] The purpose of this report is to describe an evidence-based practice (EBP) standard designed to decrease the use of restraints and seclusion of adult patients with behavioral health issues during Emergency Department (ED) visits.

The Joint Commission (TJC) and Centers for Medicare and Medicaid (CMS) recommend reducing the use of restraints and seclusion and advocating less restrictive alternatives for the patient.[1] CMS defines a restraint as "any manual method, physical or mechanical device, material, or equipment that immobilizes or reduces the ability of a patient to move his or her arms, legs, body or head freely."[3] CMS defines seclusion as "the involuntary confinement of a patient alone in a room or area from which the

Disclosures: None.
Emergency Department, The Queen's Medical Center, 1301 Punchbowl Street, Honolulu, HI 96813, USA
E-mail address: rcolehawaii@yahoo.com

Nurs Clin N Am 49 (2014) 371–381
http://dx.doi.org/10.1016/j.cnur.2014.05.010
0029-6465/14/$ – see front matter © 2014 Elsevier Inc. All rights reserved.

patient is physically prevented from leaving. Seclusion may only be used for the management of violent or self-destructive behavior."[3]

The goal for both CMS and TJC is to protect patients' basic rights, ensure patient safety, and eliminate the inappropriate use of restraints or seclusion. This is evident by the current standards in the TJC Provision of Care chapter PC.03.05.01 thru PC.03.05.11.[4] Hospitals are also required to report to CMS deaths of patients from restraint use.[4] Documentation must be included in a patient's chart, as outlined in detail by both TJC and CMS, to show that there is justification and monitoring when restraints or seclusion is initiated.[4] Examples of required documentation include clinical justification, less-restrictive alternatives tried, patient education on discontinuation criteria, and monitoring every 15 minutes for psychological status, behavior, and physical comfort.

EVIDENCE FOR PRACTICE IMPROVEMENT

The Iowa Model of Evidence-Based Practice was used to guide this EBP project (**Box 1**).[5]

TRIGGERS

This project took place in an acute-care medical center accredited by TJC. The facility is a level 2 trauma center, licensed for 505 acute beds and 28 subacute beds, and widely known for programs in behavioral medicine, emergency medicine, and other areas including cancer, cardiovascular disease, and neuroscience. The medical center is the only one in Hawaii to have achieved Magnet status, the highest institutional honor for nursing and patient care excellence, from the American Nurses Credentialing Center.

The ED sees more than 60,000 patients per year and approximately 10% (15–20 patients per day) have at least 1 behavioral health issue. Many of these patients are brought in directly by the city police department for a psychiatric evaluation because they are considered to be dangerous to themselves or others. In some cases, these patients are in an altered mental state caused by drugs, alcohol, or psychosis, and have tried to assault staff or attempted to hurt themselves or others. Managing the behavior in these types of patients can be challenging. In some situations, individuals exhibiting extremely violent or aggressive behaviors are placed in restraints or seclusion as an initial intervention for patient and staff safety.

Box 1
Summary of the Iowa model of steps
Identify triggers
Priority topic for the organization
Form a team
Assemble literature
Critique and synthesize
Pilot the change
Institute the change
Monitor the outcome
Disseminate the results

ORGANIZATIONAL PRIORITY

In 2011, the Medical Center's Restraint Committee developed a goal to reduce restraint use throughout the organization to zero. The ED was tasked with determining the best practice for managing violent or aggressive behaviors of patients seen in the ED with the goal of reducing the use of restraints and seclusion. This was a daunting task because of the high volume of patients exhibiting violent and agitated behaviors seen in the ED daily.

FORMING A TEAM

A team leader was identified and recruited staff that could function as opinion leaders who are respected and influential among peers. Unit change champions, an advance practice nurse as the clinical expert, and a manger were also asked to join the team. Once the team was formed, a charter was created, and members committed to meeting monthly for the duration of the project, estimated to be around 2 years. The final team included ED nurses, a psychiatric aide, ED clinical operations managers, a clinical nurse specialist, and a performance improvement (PI) coordinator. Emergency and psychiatric attending physicians were consulted ad hoc on a regular basis for their feedback.

ASSEMBLE RELEVANT LITERATURE

A literature search was conducted using Pub Med, CINAHL, Google scholar, and EBSCO Host. Search terms included *restraints*, *seclusion*, *managing agitation*, *emergency*, and *behavioral health*. Only 6 relevant articles were found initially, because most articles pertained to the inpatient setting. We tried different search terms and finally ended up with 24 articles. Two to 3 articles were sent to the team members for review each month. Discussion and article critique occurred at the monthly ED Restraint Reduction Team meeting. This process of critiquing articles spanned a 1-year period. Data were kept in a literature matrix that everyone could access on a shared drive.

CRITIQUE AND SYNTHESIS OF LITERATURE

One guideline and 24 articles were reviewed, critiqued, and graded for strength of evidence using the Mosby's evidence rating scale[6–8] ranging from level I (meta-analysis) to level VII (authority opinion or expert committee reports) (**Table 1**).

Synthesis of data was done after a year of literature review. Several themes keep emerging as factors influencing the use of restraints and seclusion on agitated or violent patients. The initial plan was to develop an algorithm to determine appropriate use of restraints or seclusion. However, under the guidance of the Director of Nursing Research, it was decided that the core strategies on best practice would be used in lieu of a restraints and seclusion algorithm. The core strategies, or common themes, to reduce the use of restraints and seclusion came down to 6 major components (**Box 2**). The most significant strategies included:

1. Use of noncoercive de-escalation to engage the patient and gain their trust
2. Better understanding of staff about the wide variety of available alternatives.

Several months after completing the literature synthesis, The American Psychiatric Association published a series of articles in the *Western Journal of Emergency Medicine* for Best Practices in Evaluation and Treatment of Agitation (BETA Project). These articles proved to be an invaluable reference substantiating the best practices

Table 1 Mosby's level of evidence		
	Mosby's Level of Evidence	**Articles Reviewed**
Level I	Meta-analysis	6
Level II	Experimental design aka randomized controlled trial	
Level III	Quasi-experimental design	
Level IV	Case controlled, cohort studies, longitudinal studies	1
Level V	Correlation studies	
Level VI	Descriptive studies including • Surveys • Cross-sectional design • Developmental design • Qualitative studies	8
Level VII	Authority opinion or expert committee reports	8
Other	PI; Review of literature.	1

From Melnyk B. A focus on adult acute and critical care. Worldviews Evid Based Nurs 2004;1(3): 194–7; with permission.

that were identified by the team.[1,9–13] The articles consolidated EBPs and expert opinion. The team found the information very similar to the core strategies that were identified during the synthesis of the data.

ANALYSIS

The team performed a gap analysis to determine the deficiencies between the evidence-based core strategies identified from the research synthesis and the current practices occurring in the ED setting. The gap analysis was determined by observation of current practice, chart review, staff feedback, and an environmental scan of the ED setting.

Practice Analysis

Practice analysis revealed that (1) staff did not use de-escalation techniques consistently as a way to engage patients exhibiting agitated or violent behaviors, and (2) alternatives to restraints and seclusion were not always considered or attempted before using the more restrictive methods of restraints and seclusion. Typically, patients exhibiting agitation were immediately placed in restraints or seclusions,

---

Box 2
Core strategies to reduce use of restraints and seclusion

1. Leadership support and commitment
2. Environment ensures safety. Physical setting is safe for patient and staff.
3. Change culture by understanding the trauma-informed care practice model and patient rights. The use of restraints or seclusion is considered a treatment failure.
4. Increase the use of verbal de-escalation and provide alternatives
5. Training of staff in concepts of primary and secondary prevention use of de-escalation techniques.
6. Data transparency and the use of data to trend practice

particularly if the staff perceived that the behaviors put the patient, staff, or others at risk for injury. Staff did not use or understand the trauma-informed care model of practice, described below, nor did they know how to use noncoercive de-escalation techniques to manage patients with violent or aggressive behaviors.

Trauma-informed care refers to the fact that most individuals seeking public behavioral health services have histories of physical and sexual abuse and other types of trauma-inducing experiences. These experiences often lead to mental health and co-occurring disorders such as substance abuse, eating disorders, and contact with the criminal justice system. Clinicians using trauma-informed care practices are cognizant that approaches to patients in an environment like the ED need to be supportive to avoid retraumatization. Health care providers recognize that service environments are often traumatizing and promote neutral, objective, and supportive language. It is important to value the individual in all aspects of care and avoid shaming or humiliation at all times. Providers should practice in a culture that presumes that every person in the treatment setting has been exposed to abuse, violence, neglect, or other traumatic experiences and take measures to avoid retraumatization.

Environment Analysis

Environment analysis included a review and examination of the physical layout of the behavioral health area in the ED in terms of safety for the agitated patient and for staff. Although the area was found to be safe, the environment was very stark and unwelcoming.

OUTCOMES TO BE ACHIEVED

Based on the findings above and the substantive information from the BETA project, it was clear that the focus needed to be on (1) changing the culture of the use of seclusion and restraints, (2) providing a therapeutic milieu for the agitated patient, and (3) increasing the use of noncoercive de-escalation techniques as ways to calm an agitated or violent patient. The goal was to use restraints or seclusion as a last resort—considering it a "treatment failure."

IMPLEMENTATION STRATEGIES
Education

ED leadership was consulted and approved development of a 4-hour training course for all staff integrating the BETA Project recommendations and cultural changes toward decreasing restraint use, verbal de-escalation techniques, alternatives to restraints, and pharmacologic strategies to decrease seclusion and restraint utilization (**Table 2**). The class was entitled Management of the Agitated Patient in the Emergency Department. The long-range plan was to require it for all staff if the pilot was successful.

Pilot

The 4-hour training class was piloted in February 2012 with 2 new-to-specialty nurses and 4 new graduate nurses who enrolled in the ED core orientation course. Participants were required to read 2 of the BETA Project articles and complete homework before attending the workshop. The workshop included didactic simulations created by staff, and role play was used to reinforce key concepts.

A posttest and class evaluation was completed by the pilot group. Most nurses who attended the course found the content and didactic simulation activities valuable and something they could easily integrate into their current practice. Curriculum for the

Table 2		
Class syllabus for management of the agitated patient in the ED		
Time	**Topic**	**Objectives/Content**
0700–0745 45 min	Introduction	Review worksheet Regulatory-patient safety, patient rights. EPB based on IOWA Model Trauma-informed care
0745–0815 20 min	Med/Psych Evaluation	Review best practices in evaluation and triage of agitated patient in terms of medical & psych evaluation (using the EBP treatment algorithm for triage)
0815–0900 45 min	De-escalation techniques	
0900–0915 15 min	Break	
0915–1000 45 min	Alternatives to seclusions and restraints	Review EBP alternative therapies to seclusion & restraints Brief overview of pharmacology
1000–1100	Staff safety & simulation activity	Review staff safety in management of agitated patient
1100–1130	Posttest & evaluation	Participants complete posttest, active participation in evaluation/discussion

course was revised in 2013 based on feedback, requesting more psychopharmacology and additional didactic simulations.

ED leadership was consulted regarding scheduling the class on a monthly basis to accommodate the large number of staff in the department. The team quickly realized that not involving ED leadership in the curriculum creation and roll-out phase was an important omission in the process. ED leadership felt strongly that it was important for ED staff to have the mandatory housewide Crisis Prevention course first before taking the Management of the Agitated Patient in the Emergency Department Class. The Crisis Prevention class is a housewide course for all hospital staff but not specific for ED situations. The team is exploring a collaborative process to integrate these 2 classes into a 1-day training seminar for ED staff.

Environment

To improve the physical layout of the department, furniture was changed, rooms were painted lavender to reflect a more soothing environment, and a chalk board was installed for patients. An occupational therapist was consulted to discuss alternatives that could be used such as weighted blankets and CD players for those patients who required extended stays in the behavioral health area in the ED while awaiting admission or medical clearance. The CD players were a distraction and provided music for relaxation.

DATA

Transparency of restraint and seclusion data was a core strategy to reducing restraints. An operational report was created to monitor restraint and seclusion hours and number of patient episodes. Base line data were obtained and updated monthly. These data were posted on the ED Web site, shared in huddles, discussed at unit council meetings, and presented at ED leadership meetings. These data were also presented at the hospitalwide restraint committee meeting and served as a metric for monitoring the success of the project. Results were also presented at the Pacific Institute Nursing Research Conference (PIN) as a poster session in 2012.

Documentation Audits

The ED PI Coordinator developed a monitoring tool and instructed a clinical ladder nurse on the team to perform monthly chart audits on all patients that had been restrained or placed in seclusion. A Restraint Nursing-Sensitive Indicator calculation, using the monthly data, was created with an internal benchmark. Nursing-sensitive indicators are required for all Magnet hospital departments to measure nursing-specific outcomes. There was no available indicator or national benchmark, so the following formula used total number of hours that ED patients were in seclusion or restraints divided by the total number of patient behavioral health hours in the ED multiplied by 1000. A target goal of 0.13 was established, because our baseline data showed that we were around 0.20.

Example formula:

$$\frac{\text{Total time ED behavioral health pts were in restraints or seclusion}}{\text{Total ED behavioral health patient hours}} \times 1000$$

Data Collection

Data collection of the Restraint Nursing-Sensitive Indicator data, number of episodes, and restraint and seclusion hours began in July 2011 and continued until September 2013. An episode was any time a restraint or seclusion was started and stopped on a patient. There were some patients who had 2 episodes during the same ED visit. Eight quarters of data are required and reported for Magnet hospitals. Monthly chart audits were reviewed with individual staff to provide them with feedback and used as "teachable moments," reinforcing the use of de-escalation techniques.

EVALUATION
Staff

The 4-hour class has been held twice and is scheduled for all future ED staff and new-to-specialty ED classes. Evaluations from staff who have attended the class are positive, and staff report that content and simulations have helped them feel more comfortable with de-escalation techniques and using alternative therapies for interacting with the agitated patient in the ED behavioral health area.

Number of Episodes

An episode starts when restraints are applied or the patient is placed in seclusion. The episode ends when all restraints have been removed or the patient is no longer in seclusion. An analysis of data from monthly audits found that there were fewer episodes of restraint use and seclusion from July 2011 to September 2013 (**Fig. 1**). Initially, there were 15 to 20 episodes per month, which decreased to no episodes in September 2013. Staff members are implementing less restrictive alternatives (eg, de-escalation, redirecting patients, creating a therapeutic relationship) and are more aware of the importance of decreasing restraint use unless patient or staff safety is jeopardized.

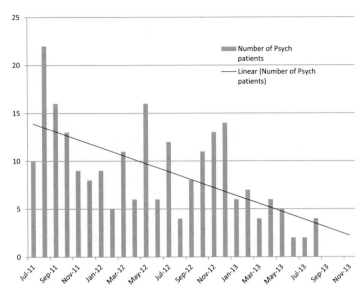

Fig. 1. Number of ED behavioral health patients restrained or secluded.

Restraint/Seclusion Hours

The time the restraint is applied or the patient is placed in seclusion to the time the restraint is removed or seclusion ends equals the hours in seclusion or restraint. All of the hours are added to equal the total number of hours over 1 month in which restraints or seclusion was used in the ED. Overall ED behavioral health seclusion and restraint hours were reduced from 38.5 h/mo in August 2011 to 0 h/mo in September 2013 (**Fig. 2**). Episode duration is shorter overall, and documentation

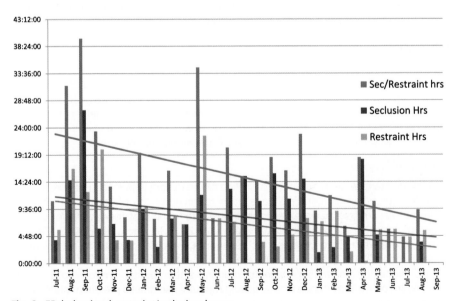

Fig. 2. ED behavioral restraint/seclusion hours.

compliance is much better. Seclusion was also found to be used more frequently than restraints, because it is a less-restrictive intervention opposed to restraints.

Restraint Nursing-Sensitive Indicator

At the start of the data collection period (August–September 2011), the initial Restraint Nursing-sensitive Indicator increased to 0.20 with a subsequent steady decline to 0.0 in September of 2013 (**Fig. 3**). These data support BETA Project best practices to use noncoercive de-escalation with the goal being to calm agitated patients and gain their cooperation in the evaluation and treatment of the agitation. Changing the culture through staff understanding of trauma-informed care, acknowledging patient rights, and providing staff training in concepts of primary and secondary prevention were keys in improving the patient outcomes.

LESSONS LEARNED
Leadership

There were several key learning opportunities during the 2-year implementation of this evidence-based project. One lesson learned was the importance of consistent team membership. The project team was initially supported by an ED manager who left within 6 months. A second ED manager joined the team but left within the year when a third manager joined the team. This change in ED leadership caused delays in project implementation as new managers learned about the EBP and provided variable support for scheduling and approving the 4-hour ED class. Having a consistent manager throughout the process would have been ideal.

Analysis

Synthesis of the literature and management of the literature matrix also provided the team with several challenges. The team read 24 articles and had difficulty interpreting all of the information, quality evidence, and best practices. Although articles had been graded by levels of evidence, many articles did not provide the relevant evidence needed to provide a research foundation for project implementation. Consultation with the Director of Nursing Research provided direction in consolidating and summarizing recurring themes into core strategies, allowing the team to develop a plan.

With regard to organizing the literature into an evidence matrix, it was helpful to have everyone enter their own literature review information and have one individual monitor to make sure it was kept up to date. To support this process, a shared drive was

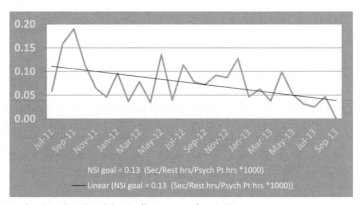

Fig. 3. Restraint Nursing-Sensitive Indicator; goal = 0.13.

created for the project so that all members could access the matrix at their convenience. During meetings in which articles were collectively reviewed and critiqued, one team member was designated as matrix scribe.

Data Transparency

Sharing restraint practice data trends was highly effective. Staff knew that restraint hours were being monitored and that results were being shared throughout the organization. As improvements were made, staff members became invested in the project's success and were increasingly committed to implementing the practice changes. Sharing positive results at housewide restraint meetings showed that restraint use could be decreased and set an example for other departments.

Stakeholder

Key stakeholder involvement in process change is critically important. Once the behavioral health department learned of the new class for the ED, they wanted to provide support to the team by understanding the content of the class and volunteering to assist by teaching the de-escalation session. The Behavioral Health Department support provided expertise in strategies for managing patient agitation. The behavioral health staff was also willing to work with the ED team to update the content in the housewide class to help meet the training needs of ED staff. The courses continue to be revised through collaboration between the ED and the Behavioral Health Departments as this project continues.

Providers

One area in which improvement was needed was encouraging more engagement with ED providers. It became clear that provider involvement was needed during medical screening examinations and the initial treatment of the agitated patient. Traditionally, the hospital's providers may turn to sedation or restraints as the first-line treatment of an agitated patient to protect them from harming themselves or the staff. Provider feedback about alternative therapies as first-line therapies would have helped increase staff awareness and may have led to greater provider buy-in for the practice change.

SUMMARY

Evidence supports reducing the use of restraints and seclusion because these episodes can result in psychological harm or physical injury to patients and staff. The goal was to discover better, more therapeutic methods for managing agitated ED behavioral health patients to minimize the use of restraints and seclusion. Training in verbal de-escalation techniques and simulation practice were key strategies in providing the staff with the necessary tools and knowledge to change their practice to one of trauma-informed care.

Staff exposure to less-restrictive alternatives helped increase staff awareness of these strategies. The opportunity to use alternatives that are available, such as redirection, weighted blankets, active listening, soothing communication style, reality links, and a quiet room, gave the staff access to new tools and therapies. The use of these alternatives has allowed staff to successfully avoid the more restrictive interventions.

The culture in the ED has changed from reflexively applying restraints or using seclusion with an agitated patient to using noncoercive de-escalation techniques and attempting to develop a therapeutic relationship with the patient. Engaging the patient in dialogue and developing a therapeutic relationship are skills that can be learned with practice. ED staff members now think of restraints and seclusion as treatment failures and feel proud when they have successfully kept the patient out of restraints. This is a very rewarding feeing in the complex world of emergency medicine. This new culture allows staff to avoid the physical and psychological trauma to patients and staff by practicing what was learned through this evidenced-based process.

REFERENCES

1. Knox DK, Holloman GH Jr. Use and avoidance of seclusion and restraint: consensus statement of the American Association for Emergency Psychiatry Project Beta Seclusion and Restraint Workgroup. West J Emerg Med 2012;13: 35–40.
2. Mohr WK, Petti TA, Mohr BD. Adverse effects associated with physical restraint. Can J Psychiatry 2003;48:330–7.
3. Department of Health and Human Services. Conditions of participation: patient rights. Fed Regist 2008;482(13):A0159–62, A0185–7.
4. The Joint Commission. Hospital Accreditation Standards. 2014: provision of care, treatment, and services Chapter PC1-70.
5. Titler MG, Kleiber C, Rakel B, et al. The Iowa model of evidenced-based practice to promote quality care. Crit Care Nurs Clin North Am 2001;13:497–509.
6. Melnyk BM. A focus on adult acute and critical care. Worldviews Evid Based Nurs 2004;1(3):194–7.
7. Guyatt G, Rennie D. User's guides to the medical literature. Washington, DC: American Medical Association Press; 2002.
8. Harris RP, Helfand M, Woolf SH, et al. Current methods of the US preventive services taskforce. A review of the process. Am J Prev Med 2001; 20(Suppl 3):21–5.
9. Holloman G, Zeller S. Overview of project BETA: best practices in evaluation and treatment of agitation. West J Emerg Med 2012;13:1–2.
10. Nordstrom K, Zun L, Wilson M, et al. Medical evaluation and triage of the agitated patent: consensus statement of the American Association for Emergency Psychiatry Project BETA Medical Evaluation Workgroup. West J Emerg Med 2012;13:2–10.
11. Stowell K, Florence P, Harman H, et al. Psychiatric evaluation of the agitated patient: consensus statement of the American Association for Emergency Psychiatry Project BETA Psychiatric Evaluation Workgroup. West J Emerg Med 2012;13:11–6.
12. Richmond J, Berlin J, Fishkind A, et al. Verbal de-escalation of the agitated patient: consensus statement of the American Association for Emergency Psychiatry Project BETA De-escalation Workgroup. West J Emerg Med 2012; 13:17–25.
13. Wilson M, Pepper D, Currier G, et al. The psychopharmacology of agitation: consensus statement of the American Association for Emergency Psychiatry Project BETA Psychopharmacology Workgroup. West J Emerg Med 2012;13: 26–34.

Promoting Sleep in the Adult Surgical Intensive Care Unit Patients to Prevent Delirium

Rose K.L. Hata, MS, RN, APRN, CCRN, CCNS[a],*, Lois Han, BSN, RN, CCRN[a],
Jill Slade, BSN, RN, CCRN[a], Asa Miyahira, BSN, RN, CCRN[a],
ChristyAnne Passion, MSN, RN, CCRN[a], Maimona Ghows, MD[a],
Kara Izumi, PharmD, BCPS, BCNSP[a], Mihae Yu, MD[b]

KEYWORDS

- Surgical intensive care unit • Sleep management • Evidence-based practice
- Nonpharmacologic delirium prevention

KEY POINTS

- Ensuring adequate sleep for hospitalized patients is important for reducing stress, improving healing, and decreasing episodes of delirium.
- The purpose of this project was to implement a Sleep Program for stable patients in the surgical intensive care unit, thereby changing sleep management practices and ensuring quality of care using an evidence-based practice approach.
- Improving patient satisfaction with sleep by 28 percentage points may be attributed to a standardized process of providing a healing environment for patients to sleep.

INTRODUCTION

Sleep is important for the healing process, yet sleep deprivation in acutely ill patients remains a common issue in hospitals.[1–3] Physical illness, emotional stress, environmental change, nonoptimal lighting, and high environmental noise are factors that can cause sleep deprivation in hospitalized patients.[4] Creating a quiet hospital environment is one component to promoting and improving the quality of sleep for

Funding: This project was partially funded by the Agency for Healthcare Research & Quality, 5R13HS017892; Hawaii State Center for Nursing; and Queen Emma Nursing Institute, The Queen's Medical Center, Honolulu, HI.
[a] SICU, The Queen's Medical Center, 1301 Punchbowl Street, Honolulu, HI 96813, USA;
[b] Surgical Critical Care Fellowship, Department of Surgery, The Queen's Medical Center, University of Hawaii, 1356 Lusitana Street, 6th Floor, Honolulu, HI 96813, USA
* Corresponding author.
E-mail address: rhata@queens.org

hospitalized patients.[5] The World Health Organization (WHO) recommends sound levels of less than 30 to 40 dB for hospital rooms, which is equivalent to quiet whispers in the library.[6,7]

Providing a restful environment is particularly challenging for the intensive care unit (ICU) setting. ICUs by nature are noisy places where equipment frequently alarms. Constant nursing and medical interventions make uninterrupted sleep almost impossible. Patients in the ICU, because of their medical acuity and decreased ability to cope with stress, are at a higher risk for delirium, a condition aggravated by sleep deprivation. As much as 73% of surgical ICU (SICU) patients may be affected by delirium.[8] Delirium is associated with an increase in mortality and length of stay in the hospital.[9,10] In addition, patients who develop delirium in the ICU may have cognitive impairment for up to 1 year after hospitalization.[11]

Despite the inherent difficulties, creating a quiet environment in the ICU could benefit this patient population and positively affect delirium rates. The purpose of this article is to describe the effect of an evidence-based nonpharmacologic nursing guideline for sleep management for stable SICU patients using the Iowa Model of Evidence-Based Practice to Promote Quality Care (**Box 1**).[12]

Triggers

Patients' hospital experiences, including their perception of a quiet environment at night, are measured through Hospital Consumer Assessment of Healthcare Providers and Systems (HCAHPS) surveys. Patient perception survey results are reported publicly. The US Government uses these data as a quality indicator to determine hospital reimbursement rates.[13] Hospitals strive to achieve an "always" rating on all scales to receive optimal reimbursement. Medicare's quarterly report from 2013 revealed that an average of 60% of patients across the United States reported the area around their hospital room was "always" quiet at night. By comparison, patients in the State of Hawaii reported that their hospital room was "always" quiet 56% of the time; the site of this project, a major tertiary hospital, averaged "always" quiet only 53% of the time.[14]

Box 1
Steps of project using the Iowa model

Steps of the project were as follows:

1. Triggers (problem focused and/or knowledge focused)
2. Organizational priority (is this topic a priority for the organization?)
3. Form a team
4. Assemble relevant research and related articles
5. Critique and synthesize research
6. Determine outcomes to be achieved
7. Baseline data
8. Design the EBP guideline
9. Implement EBP
10. Evaluate process and outcomes
11. Modify the practice guidelines
12. Institute the change in practice

Abbreviation: EBP, evidence-based practice.

This project took place in the SICU of an acute-care medical facility accredited by The Joint Commission. The facility is licensed for 505 acute beds and 28 subacute beds, and is widely known for its programs in cancer, cardiovascular disease, neuroscience, orthopedics, surgery, emergency medicine and trauma, and behavioral medicine. The hospital is the only one in the State to have achieved Magnet status, the highest institutional honor for hospital excellence, from the American Nurses Credentialing Center. Magnet recognition is held by less than 6% of hospitals in the United States.

Clinicians are aware of the importance of sleep for patients. However, multiple interventions and tasks needed to care for the critically ill SICU patient make it difficult to provide an environment conducive to sleep. A structured Sleep Program fosters a culture whereby quality sleep time can be provided for patients.[15,16] In the SICU at the author's tertiary hospital, sleep promotion for ICU patients is particularly challenging because of frequent nursing interventions, high noise levels related to clinical alarms, medical equipment, and staff conversations. Disruption of the sleep/wake cycle can interfere with healing and may contribute to delirium in the SICU patient.[17] This SICU lacked a culture of prioritizing sleep for the critically ill patients on a consistent basis.

Organizational Priority

Delirium prevention in the ICU was a key priority for the organization. Because sleep disturbances contribute to delirium, the organization and the unit leaders embraced implementation of the Sleep Program. The SICU leadership's support of this program was evidenced by the amount of resources and time that was provided in staff education. Over a period of 5 months, a delirium curriculum (a series of interactive courses) was provided to all SICU nurses, including (1) Delirium 101: Introduction to delirium; (2) Delirium 201: Assessing delirium; and (3) Delirium 301: Pharmacologic management of pain, agitation, and delirium (PAD).

The Delirium 101 course was conducted by one of the expert SICU staff nurses. This course focused on updating the staff on the current literature in delirium and emphasizing the improvement opportunities in the unit. This course set the tone and case for action for other upcoming series. Delirium 201 reviewed how clinicians can influence patient outcomes by systematically assessing for delirium on all patients. This course focused on learning the Confusion Assessment Method for the ICU (CAM-ICU), and emphasized both pharmacologic and nonpharmacologic recommendations for managing PAD. Delirium 301 classes were conducted by the SICU pharmacist and concentrated on review of frequently used medications for PAD management.

After completion of the 3 courses, the Sleep Program was introduced in the SICU. Having the delirium curriculum first was strategic to moving toward promoting sleep, and helped the staff become receptive to the Sleep Program.

Formation of a Team

A multidisciplinary SICU evidence-based practice (EBP) team was formed to promote sleep in the ICU as one approach to preventing delirium. Team members included staff nurses, the nurse manager, the clinical nurse specialist, EBP mentors, the ICU pharmacist, and a physician champion. Some members of this SICU EBP team were also members of other interdisciplinary hospital teams managing PAD (**Fig. 1**).

Members of the SICU EBP team updated and sought feedback from the SICU nursing unit council on a routine basis. The SICU physician leaders were also frequently updated and were intimately involved in the development of the Sleep Program.

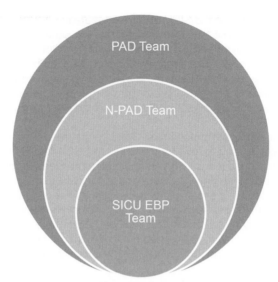

Fig. 1. Team structures. Surgical Intensive Care Unit Evidence-Based Practice (SICU EBP) Team: The team consisted of staff nurses, nurse manager, clinical nurse specialist, EBP mentors, ICU pharmacist, and a physician champion. This unit based interdisciplinary team focused on delirium prevention in the SICU, including developing the SICU Sleep Program. Nursing Pain, Agitation, and Delirium (N-PAD) Team: The team consisted of nursing representatives from all ICUs at the hospital, and representatives from rehabilitation and respiratory therapy departments. The goals of this team were to standardize EBP and other PAD-related projects while focusing on nonpharmacologic interventions. PAD Team: The team consisted of intensivists, pharmacists, nurse managers, educator, and clinical nurse specialists from all ICUs at the hospital. This interdisciplinary leadership team provided oversight on managing PAD based on Society of Critical Care Medicine PAD guidelines[9], including pharmacologic interventions.

EVIDENCE FOR PRACTICE IMPROVEMENT
Assemble Relevant Research

The SICU EBP team initially assembled relevant research and literature to prevent delirium in the SICU. The team spent more than 9 months reviewing articles on prevention of delirium in the ICU. Among many nonpharmacologic recommendations to prevent delirium, the team concluded that sleep promotion may be difficult to attain and yet remain important in the ICU.

After the initial review of the literature, the team concentrated on best practices on providing sleep for the SICU patients in order to reduce delirium. The literature search was done using CINAHL and Medline databases for articles from the past 10 years. Key search words included "sleep promotion," "sleep deprivation," "critical care," "quiet time," "noise reduction," "delirium prevention," and "intensive care unit." More than 40 articles and one clinical guideline were reviewed and critiqued. Of these articles, 13 recent ones were specific to sleep promotion in the ICU **(Table 1)**.

Critique and Synthesize Research

According to the 2013 clinical guideline for successfully managing PAD, the Society of Critical Care Medicine (SCCM) continues to strongly recommend affecting ICU outcomes by promoting sleep in adult ICU patients.[9] SCCM supports interventions

Table 1
Levels of articles reviewed

Mosby Level	Description	No. of Articles on Nursing Interventions (Sleep Promotion; Noise Levels; Quiet Time)	No. of Articles on Sedation Management/ Delirium
I	Meta-analysis	—	1
II	Experimental design (RCT)	—	8
III	Quasi-experimental design	—	1
IV	Case-controlled, cohort studies, longitudinal studies	1	7
V	Correlation studies	1	—
VI	Descriptive studies including surveys, cross-sectional design, developmental design, qualitative studies	1	10
VII	Authority opinion or expert committee reports	1	1
Other	Performance improvement; Review of literature	9	6
	Practice guideline	1	

Abbreviation: RCT, randomized controlled trial.

such as music therapy, sleep, and relaxation to minimize, prevent, and treat PAD. These interventions can decrease heart rate, respiratory rate, myocardial oxygen demand, and anxiety.[2,9]

To optimize sleep promotion, clinicians need to be mindful of a healing environment from the patient's perspective.[5] By promoting activities during the day, natural and adequate sleep at night can be provided. Natural sleep cues (such as lighting and noise) also help to promote sleep. It is best to avoid frequent waking tasks and to prevent interruptions. Staff conversation and alarms are generally regarded as the most disturbing noises for sleep in the ICU.[18] For continuity of promoting sleep, all interventions need to be tailored and specific to the patient's plan of care. Every critically ill patient may not be allotted optimal sleep time because of the care interventions necessary to the medical management of the ICU patient.[17]

The literature emphasized that sleep is an essential component of healing because lack of sleep impairs tissue repair and increases levels of physiologic stress.[4] Quality sleep requires a minimum increment of 90 minutes of uninterrupted sleep.[19] To provide environments conducive to sleep, some ICUs have implemented 2-hour "quiet times" during the day and at night, and have observed that these intentional periods help promote sleep for patients while allowing nurses to catch up with documentation and other tasks.[15,17]

To provide an optimal resting period, it is important to solicit patient preferences for the patient's optimal sleep environment. For example, intentional actions such as closing room doors for noise control without involving the patients may lead to some patients having feelings of isolation or higher anxiety levels. Moreover, direct nursing observation of patient sleep may not be as accurate as directly asking the patients regarding their quality of sleep. Engaging patients in the evaluation of their sleep is an effective way to evaluate their sleep quality.[5]

IMPLEMENTATION STRATEGIES
Outcomes to be Achieved

This project concentrated on the quality of patients' sleep. The aim of the SICU Sleep Program was to identify patients who were stable enough to be uninterrupted at night from midnight to 4 AM. The goals were to: (1) increase patients' ability to sleep, (2) increase patients' reports of feeling rested, and (3) address barriers to sleep as identified by patients.

Baseline Data

Before the Sleep Program, baseline data were collected from 10 "stable" SICU patients who would have qualified for the Sleep Program. Of the 10 patients, 50% reported that they were able to sleep and 50% that they felt rested. Noise, interruptions by staff, pain, and fear were the reported barriers to sleep and feeling rested.

Design the EBP Guideline

Integrating key concepts from the literature to design a successful SICU Sleep Program, the team developed a standardized process of providing sleep for the stable SICU patients (**Box 2**). Because the standard routine care for these patients included hourly intake/output monitoring and vital-sign assessment at least every 2 hours, a standardized physician order was created for stable patients (**Box 3**). For the Sleep Program to be effective, all relevant hospital disciplines had to align with the plan. It was important for the nurses and respiratory therapists to change their workflow so that tasks such as bathing, tubing changes, and dressing changes could be streamlined at night.

Implement EBP

Finding the balance between critically managing patients and allowing uninterrupted time for sleep is challenging, especially during the acute stabilization period for ICU patients. For example, there were concerns that providing a 4-hour block of uninterrupted sleep might be inappropriate for ICU patients. Thus, it was important for the unit to define the "stable" status of the patient (**Box 4**). In addition, all patients meeting the stable status were not automatically enrolled into the Sleep Program. Instead, patients meeting the stability criteria triggered discussions during the multidisciplinary rounds whereby team members evaluated the appropriateness of the Sleep Program for each patient.

The Sleep Program proposal was presented to physicians, nurses, the unit council, and respiratory therapy department. This preliminary period of involving and explaining to stakeholders the intent and design of the proposed program, while soliciting suggestions for improvement, was crucial for clinician engagement. It also helped the EBP team to design a program that would be a good fit for the unit. Stakeholder discussions led to creative brainstorming and questions such as:

- Did we communicate the new process with all affected departments such as radiology and laboratory?
- How can patient safety be assured during the implementation of the Sleep Program?
- What do we do for "stable" patients who have pressure ulcers?

The feedback and questions helped the team to design a successful Sleep Program. Hence, other disciplines and departments (ie, radiology, and laboratory) were contacted regarding this new program.

Box 2
SICU sleep program plan: creating a standardized process

ASSESSMENT (PM shift to AM shift)

- For vented patients: RT to discuss criteria (P/F ratio)/concerns with RN
- PM shift RN to discuss patient's quality of sleep with AM shift RN

1. Provide assessments
2. Provide recommendations

DURING DAY:

1. AM shift: RN discusses sleep during multidisciplinary rounds
    a. If meeting criteria, RN consults with MD for sleep program order
    b. If MD agrees, MD writes sleep order (use template order)
    c. Add sleep section on the daily goals tool to help facilitate discussion
        i. Review effectiveness/recommendation of sleep program
        ii. List criteria for sleep program/criteria met? Yes/No
2. AM shift RN promotes patient activities during day (OT/PT, OOB, ROM, mobility, and so forth)
3. AM shift RN to consult PharmD for medication time changes, if applicable
4. AM shift RN to initiate routine tasks, as time permits (eg, baths, tubing changes, and so forth)

After ORDER (PM shift):

1. Tasks should be coordinated around the sleep time
    a. Charge nurses/other nurses to help out with various tasks such as:
        i. Baths
        ii. Intravenous tubing changes
        iii. Dressing changes
    b. Integrate into huddles: who is on the sleep program
2. Before interventions, RN must explain the following benefits of sleep to the patient (required):
    a. Promote healing
    b. Prevent confusion from lack of sleep
    c. Regulate day/night wake cycle
3. On understanding from patient, RN provides following intervention (checklist):
    a. Check alarm limits and individualize to patient as appropriate
    b. Remove glucometer from room for midnight quality check (to prevent disturbing patient)
    c. Seek patient preference for the following interventions:
        i. Turn off television (optional: low-volume music channel)
        ii. Turn off lights (optional: dimmed lights)
        iii. Close curtains[a]
        iv. Close door[a]
    d. Provide call bell within reach
        i. Visual check of patients should be done at least every hour
        ii. Sleep sign on the door (visual cue that the patient is on sleep program)

e. Other:

    i. Intravenous pumps can be placed on dim/night mode

    ii. Room sweep (eg, is volume to be infused setting adequate? Troubleshoot A-line: if needed, place arm board)

    iii. Keep voice volume to whisper in other areas, including nursing station

4. Nursing note: evaluation of the sleep program

    a. PM shift RN utilizes the template to write note

        i. Intervention

        ii. Assessment of patient

        iii. Recommendation

    b. PM shift RN "completes" order from electronic medical record

5. Cycle repeats. Sleep program order is reevaluated on a daily basis as long as the patient continues to meet criteria

    a. Return sleep sign to designated area

    b. Encourage activity (PT/OT/ROM/mobility) during day

    c. Set activity goals with patients

Abbreviations: MD, medical doctor; OOB, out of bed; OT, occupational therapy; PharmD, pharmacy doctor; PT, physical therapy; RN, registered nurse; ROM, range of motion; RT, respiratory therapist.

[a] Seeking preference is important to prevent feelings of isolation/neglect.

Tailoring the program to each patient was equally important. The Sleep Program order was adjusted to include continuous monitoring and frequent visual checks of the patient. Nurses were empowered to interrupt the Sleep Program with any patient status changes that required nursing or medical interventions. In addition, the criteria for patients who qualified for the Sleep Program were fine-tuned. Because the status of the ICU patients may frequently change, the Sleep Program order was valid for one night, with re-evaluation daily for appropriate use of the program. The wound care Clinical Nurse Specialist was consulted regarding safety and efficacy of those patients who might be at high risk for pressure ulcers. Patients were carefully monitored and evaluated daily for possible pressure ulcer issues. By being vigilant and proactive in repositioning the patients as necessary, the Sleep Program did not have a negative impact on pressure ulcers.

Before the rollout, clinicians were educated on the importance of promoting sleep as a strategy for preventing delirium. To aid the program, a checklist of nursing

Box 3
Standardized physician order

ICU Sleep Program order:

Do not disturb the patient from 0000 to 0400, including not performing routine vital signs. The primary RN may interrupt this program with patient condition changes.

Continue to monitor and document electrocardiogram, respiratory rate, oxygen saturation, and so forth from central monitor. Perform visual checks of patients at least hourly.

For patients with pressure ulcers, continue to turn patients every 2 hours during the sleep program.

Box 4
Definition of stable SICU patient

- Adult ($\geq$18 years old)
- Patient is hemodynamically stable as defined below:
  - ○ Off of all vasoactive drips
  - ○ Adequate tissue perfusion as evidenced by Oxygen Challenge Test procedure[a]
  - ○ If patient is on ventilator:
    - ■ Not on specialty ventilator such as HFOV
    - ■ PEEP less than 10
    - ■ P/F ratio greater than 250

Abbreviations: HFOV, high-frequency oscillation ventilation; PEEP, positive end-expiratory pressure.
  [a] Oxygen Challenge Test is a noninvasive method for monitoring microvascular perfusion of internal organs (ie, early detection of shock) because the skin is the first tissue bed to vasoconstrict in shock and the last to reperfuse with resuscitation.[20]

---

interventions was developed, which included a guideline to ask the patients their preference on how to best create an environment comfortable for sleeping, such as door closure, curtains drawn, lights turned off, and television tuned to white noise or turned off (**Box 5**). A poster board was developed to help educate the staff on this process (**Fig. 2**). Highly visible signs for patient rooms were developed so that others would not enter the rooms unnecessarily.

In addition to the standardized order for physicians, a nursing note template was created for nurses to evaluate the Sleep Program (**Box 6**). The Sleep Program evaluation notes contained 3 specific questions to ask the patients each morning following implementation of the Sleep Program:

1. Were you able to sleep?
2. Do you feel rested?
3. If not feeling rested, what were the barriers?

The evaluation notes also triggered the nurse to document nursing assessments and recommendations to better promote sleep for the patient. To remind clinicians about discussing the effect of the Sleep Program and/or to assess appropriateness of the program for the patient, the Sleep Program was integrated into the daily goals worksheet for discussion during daily interdisciplinary rounds.

To improve communication with other disciplines (eg, respiratory therapists, laboratory technicians, or radiology technicians) about the program, a magnet with a picture of a sheep was placed next to the room numbers of patients enrolled in the program on the magnetic assignment board (**Fig. 3**). Moreover, during shift huddles, the charge nurse notified the night shift nurses of patients who were on the Sleep Program. Charge nurses were also responsible for keeping track of patients on the Sleep Program.

EVALUATION

During the 2.5 months of the pilot, a total of 31 patients participated in the Sleep Program and 102 sleep nights were ordered. A total of 54 program evaluation notes were completed. Some evaluation notes were unavailable, owing to patient condition changes that required interruption of the Sleep Program (**Fig. 4**). Some nurses forgot

---

Box 5
SICU Sleep Program Checklist

1. Check for MD sleep order (use template for ordering Sleep Program)

2. Coordinate before sleep time/midnight:

   • Baths

   • Intravenous tubing changes

   • Dressing changes

   • VS/Assessment (2330–2359)

   • Glucose check and remove glucometer for QC

   • Room sweep: check alarm limits, dim and program VTBI on intravenous pumps

   • ETT retaping with RT

3. Explain benefits of sleep program to patient:

   • Promote healing

   • Prevent confusion from lack of sleep

   • Regulate day/night wake cycle

4. Seek patient's preferences:

   • Turn off TV or provide music channel (low volume)

   • Turn off or dim lights

   • Close curtains

   • Close door

   • Sleep sign on door

ZZZs from Midnight to 0400

Continue to monitor ECG, RR, Spo_2, and so forth from central monitor

Visual checks (of patient) hourly at central monitor

5. Coordinate after 0400:

   • VS/Assessment by RN/RT

   • AM PCXR

   • AM Labs

   • SVo_2 calibration

   • ABG

6. Evaluation:

   • Nursing progress note (use template for sleep evaluation)

   • Suggestion/Comments to oncoming shift

7. Complete Sleep Program order

Abbreviations: ABG, arterial blood gas; ECG, electrocardiogram; ETT, endotracheal tube; PCXR, portable chest x-ray; QC, quality control; RN, registered nurse; RR, respiratory rate; RT, respiratory therapist; Spo_2, oxygen saturation; SVo_2, venous oxygen saturation; VS, vital signs; VTBI, volume to be infused.

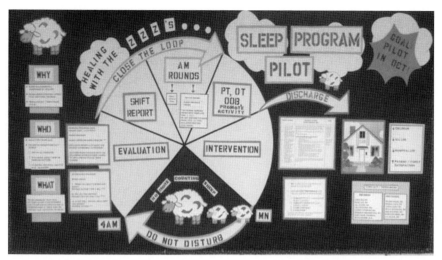

Fig. 2. Educational board for Sleep Program.

or were unaware of the use of the template note to evaluate the Sleep Program; thus, some evaluation notes were not available for analysis even though the Sleep Program order was executed.

Patients enrolled in the program reported that they were able to sleep 78% of the nights (vs 50% preimplementation) (**Fig. 5**). In addition, 69% of the time patients reported that they felt rested (vs 50% preimplementation). During the first 3 weeks of the pilot, common barriers to sleep included topics that staff could influence, such

---

Box 6
Nurse's template note on evaluating the Sleep Program in the ICU

ICU Sleep Program Note

Sleep order obtained from Dr[a]

Explained benefits of sleep to patient and patient agreeable to program.

Initiated sleep program with the following interventions: Lights/TV off, curtain pulled, door closed.

After Sleep Program

Following questions were asked to the patient:

1. Were you able to sleep last night?

Patient stated: {drop down choices: YES; NO; [a]}

2. Do you feel rested?

Patient stated: {drop down choices: YES; NO; [a]}

3. If not well rested, what kept you awake?

Patient stated: {drop down choices: [a]; Not Applicable}

RN Assessment[a]

Recommendation(s)[a]

[a] Denotes free text area by nurse.

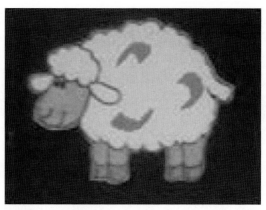

Fig. 3. Magnet with a picture of a sheep.

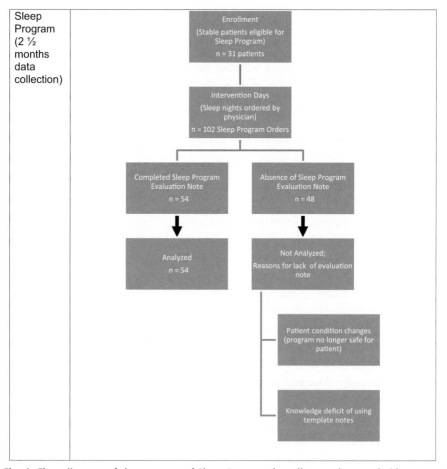

Fig. 4. Flow diagram of the progress of Sleep Program (enrollment, data analysis).

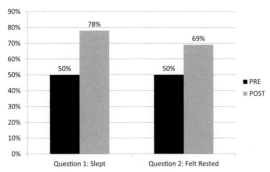

Fig. 5. Patient response data for ability to sleep and feeling rested, comparing pre-implementation and post-implementation of Sleep Program.

as laboratory sticks and noise. The most common noise reported was from clinical alarms and staff conversation. Once these common barriers had been eliminated, the common sleep barriers during the latter part of the pilot were anxiety, pain, and inability to fall asleep (**Fig. 6**). These identified and modifiable barriers were subsequently integrated into the patient's care management.

LESSONS LEARNED AND RECOMMENDATIONS FOR OTHERS

Providing quiet time for patients to sleep may sound like a simple phenomenon, but it is especially difficult in patients with critical care needs. Success of this Sleep Program can be largely attributed to targeted efforts by clinicians after emphasizing how sleep plays a vital role in the healing process.

A significant and successful strategy of the Sleep Program was to include a template evaluation note in the electronic medical record that required the nurse to evaluate the quality of a patient's sleep by directly asking the patient specific questions. In addition to important data for measuring the impact of the project, the note prompted the nurse to assess the quality of sleep.

According to Nicolas and colleagues,[21] nurses tend to overestimate the patient's perception of nighttime sleep. Involving patients in communicating their quality of sleep and identifying their own barriers and/or improvement strategies engaged both patients and staff in their care management. Moreover, this evaluation allowed the nurse to hear patient concerns directly and to appropriately tailor care to improve

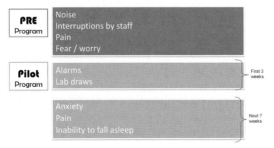

Fig. 6. Barriers identified by the patient on barriers to sleep (pre-Program, first 3 weeks of the Sleep Program, next 7 weeks of the Sleep Program).

the patient's sleep. This approach led to increased awareness in nurses that helped sustain the practice change.

As staff developed a better understanding of ICU barriers to a good night's sleep, nurses began to intervene to address the common barriers such as emotional disturbances, in particular fear and worry. Over time, the original barriers (conversations, blood draws, and so forth) were mentioned less often by patients. Nurses were reminded that they can play an important role in the healing process by meeting the emotional needs of the patients in addition to meeting physical needs.

There were barriers with the electronic evaluation note. Although it was deemed crucial in improving the patient's identified barriers for sleep, there were difficulties in accessing this template evaluation note in the electronic medical record. The restricted capability of automatic access to all users during the pilot implementation time limited the usefulness of the evaluation note and subsequent potential practice change. Although attempts were made to program all users for access, some agency and float nurses did not have ready access. Thus there was inconsistency in using the evaluation note.

Stakeholder engagement is a critical success factor. Another lesson learned was that because the Sleep Program predominantly affected the practice of nightshift clinicians, it would have been time well spent to invest more effort in engaging with these staff members early in the planning process. Recruitment of more nightshift nurses as project leaders would have been helpful.

SUMMARY

Ensuring adequate sleep for hospitalized patients is important for reducing stress, improving healing, and decreasing episodes of delirium. The purpose of this project was to implement a Sleep Program for stable SICU patients, thereby changing sleep management practices and ensuring quality of care using an EBP approach. Improving patient satisfaction with sleep by 28 percentage points may be attributed to a standardized process of providing a healing environment for patients to sleep.

ICU nurses, in particular, have the capacity to alter wake/sleep cycles and significantly improve patient outcomes by integrating nonpharmacologic interventions to promote sleep. A standardized Sleep Program raised awareness of the importance of sleep and naturally induced a quieter environment. For sustainability, direct patient feedback allowed nurses to accurately evaluate the quality of patient sleep and provide optimal conditions and advocacy for sleep.

Nurses have the ability and imperative to affect the patient's healing process by addressing barriers to sleep as identified by the patient. After removing barriers that nurses can directly influence, such as alarm noise and staff conversation, common sleep barriers for patients are related to emotional concerns. Future efforts should be directed at providing emotional support and alleviating fear during the patient's ICU stay. These additional strategies may greatly benefit the patient's quality of sleep and the healing process.

ACKNOWLEDGMENTS

The authors would like to acknowledge all SICU Staff Nurses, Physicians, Respiratory Therapists, and colleagues for their support of this project.

REFERENCES

1. Cappuccio FP, D'Elia L, Strazzullo P, et al. Sleep duration and all-cause mortality: a systematic review and meta-analysis of prospective studies. Sleep 2010;33(5):585–92.

2. Jacobi J, Fraser GL, Cousin DB, et al. Clinical practice guidelines for the sustained use of sedatives and analgesics in the critically ill adult. Crit Care Med 2002;30(1):119–41.

3. Friese RS, Diaz-Arrastia R, McBride D, et al. Quantity and quality of sleep in the surgical intensive care unit: are our patients sleeping? J Trauma 2007;63:1210–4.

4. Matthews EE. Sleep disturbances and fatigue in critically ill patients. AACN Adv Crit Care 2011;22(3):204–44.

5. Fontana CJ, Pittiglio LI. Sleep deprivation among critical care patients. Crit Care Nurs Q 2010;33(1):75–81.

6. Berglund B, Lindvall T, Schwela DH, editors. Guidelines for community noise. World Health Organization. 1999. Available at: http://www.who.int/docstore/peh/noise/guidelines2.html. Accessed July 25, 2013.

7. American Association of Audiology. Levels of noise poster. In: Turn it to the left. 2009. Available at: http://www.turnittotheleft.com/educationresources.htm. Accessed July 25, 2013.

8. Pandharipande P, Cotton BA, Shintani A, et al. Prevalence and risk factors for development of delirium in surgical and trauma intensive care unit patients. J Trauma 2008;65:34–41.

9. Barr J, Fraser GL, Puntillo K, et al. Clinical practice guidelines for the management of pain, agitation, and delirium in adult patients in the intensive care unit. Crit Care Med 2013;41:263–306.

10. Ely EW, Shintani A, Truman B, et al. Delirium as a predictor of mortality in mechanically ventilated patients in the intensive care unit. JAMA 2004;291(14):1753–62.

11. Girard T, Jackson J, Pandharipande P, et al. Delirium as a predictor of long-term cognitive impairment in survivors of critical illness. Crit Care Med 2010;38(7):1513–20.

12. Titler MG, Kleiber C, Steelman V, et al. The Iowa model of evidence-based practice to promote quality care. Crit Care Nurs Clin North Am 2001;13(4):497–509.

13. HCAHPS fact sheet, May 2012. In: HCAHPS - hospital survey. 2012. Available at: http://www.hcahpsonline.org/files/HCAHPS%20Fact%20Sheet%20May%202012.pdf. Accessed July 24, 2013.

14. Hospital profile, The Queen's Medical Center, patient survey results. In: Medicare.gov Hospital Compare. 2013. Available at: http://www.medicare.gov/hospitalcompare/profile.html#profTab=1&ID=120001&state=HI&lat=0&lng=0. Accessed July 24, 2013.

15. Dennis CM, Lee R, Woodard EK, et al. Benefits of quiet time for neuro-intensive care patients. J Neurosci Nurs 2010;42(2):217–24.

16. Lower J, Bonsack C, Guion J. Consider implementing a quiet time for patient relaxation to enhance the healing process and increase patient satisfaction. Nurs Manage 2003;34(4):40A-D.

17. Bruno JJ, Warren ML. Intensive care unit delirium. Crit Care Nurs Clin North Am 2010;22(2):161–78.

18. Gabor JY, Cooper AB, Crombach SA, et al. Contribution of the intensive care unit environment to sleep disruption in mechanically ventilated patients and healthy subjects. Am J Respir Crit Care Med 2003;167:708–15.

19. Patel M, Chipman J, Carlin BW, et al. Sleep in the intensive care unit setting. Crit Care Nurs Q 2008;31(4):309–18.

20. Yu M, Chapital A, Ho HC, et al. A prospective randomized trial comparing oxygen delivery versus transcutaneous pressure of oxygen values as resuscitation goals. Shock 2007;27(6):615–22.

21. Nicolas A, Aizpitarte E, Iruarrizaga A, et al. Perception of night-time sleep by surgical patients in an intensive care unit. Nurs Crit Care 2008;13(1):25–33.

Normothermia for NeuroProtection

It's Hot to Be Cool

Juliet G. Beniga, BSN, RN, CNRN, CCRN[a],*,
Katherine G. Johnson, MS, RN, APRN, CCRN, CNRN, CNS-BC[b],
Debra D. Mark, PhD, RN[c]

KEYWORDS

- Normothermia • NeuroProtection • Evidence • Brain injury

KEY POINTS

- Nurses are essential in the care of individuals with neurologic injury. Severe traumatic brain injury and stroke are major health problems in the United States and a common cause of disability and death.
- Fever is a significant contributor to secondary brain insult and management is a challenge for the neurocritical care team.
- The absence of standardized guidelines likely contributes to poor surveillance and under-treatment of increased temperature.

INTRODUCTION

Nurses are essential in the care of individuals with neurologic injury. Severe traumatic brain injury (TBI) and stroke are major health problems in the United States and a common cause of disability and death. In 2003, the US Centers for Disease Control and Prevention estimated that 1.5 million people sustain a TBI each year, and approximately 50,000 people die, accounting for a mortality of about 30%. At least 5.3 million Americans, have long-term needs for assistance to perform activities of daily living because of TBI-related cognitive, physical, and psychological disabilities. The direct cost of acute care, the loss of potential income, the ongoing costs of rehabilitation, and the indirect costs to the caregivers are substantial and at times not measurable.[1]

Funding Source: The Queen's Medical Center and University of Hawaii School of Nursing & Dental Hygiene Cooperative Research Partnership Grant (439381).
The authors have no additional disclosures.
a Neuroscience Institute, Neuroscience Intensive Care Unit, The Queen's Medical Center, 1301 Punchbowl Street, Honolulu, HI 96813, USA; b Neuroscience Institute, The Queen's Medical Center, 1301 Punchbowl Street, Honolulu, HI 96813, USA; c University of Hawaii at Manoa, School of Nursing & Dental Hygiene, 2528 McCarthy Mall, Webster Hall 402, Honolulu, HI 96822, USA
* Corresponding author.
E-mail addresses: julietsmail51@gmail.com; jbeniga@queens.org

Each year, about 795,000 people have a stroke, the leading cause of serious, long-term disability in the United States.[2] Stroke costs the United States an estimated $38.6 billion each year, which includes the cost of health care services, medications, and missed days of work.[3] In Hawaii, major cardiovascular disease, which includes coronary heart disease and stroke is the leading cause of death, with a statewide mortality of 45 per 100,000 deaths in 2005.[4]

Fever is a normal immunologic response to an infectious or inflammatory process; however, increased body temperature in the presence of neurologic injury can lead to secondary brain injury.[5] Hyperthermia contributes to a state of increased cerebral metabolism that, at the cellular level, may lead to ischemia, excitotoxicity, energy failure, cerebral swelling, inflammation, and neuronal death.[6] Regardless of the cause, fever can be harmful and is associated with poor outcomes, neurologic impairment, and prolonged intensive care unit (ICU) and hospital lengths of stay.[7,8] Thus, temperature management in neurologically vulnerable patients is both a prevalent challenge and a priority.

The primary treatment goal for the care of critically ill neurocritical patients is to prevent or minimize progression of brain insult for which fever is a cause. Therefore, the purpose of this project was to develop and institutionalize a standardized evidence-based practice (EBP) protocol to reduce temperature and to maintain normothermia in the neurocritical care patient population.

EVIDENCE FOR PRACTICE IMPROVEMENT

The Iowa Model of Evidence Based Practice was used as a framework to guide the process of developing a normothermia EBP guideline. The process begins with the recognition of a problem or trigger, which may be an identified practice issue or a knowledge deficit. The organizational mission and goals are explored to determine whether the problem is a priority for the organization. If addressing the practice issue is deemed a priority, a team of stakeholders, clinicians, educators, and other advocates of EBP are assembled. The next significant step is to compile, synthesize, and critique levels of the evidence relating to the practice issue. A pilot of the practice change occurs if there is sufficient evidence to support the change. Outcomes from the implementation of a practice change are monitored, evaluated, and reported for dissemination. The Iowa model provides an algorithm that highlights key decision points helpful to facilitate progression to the next step.[9]

Knowledge and Problem Triggers

Every year nearly all patients with severe TBI and a large number of patients with a stroke diagnosis are admitted to the 500-bed tertiary medical center located in the heart of downtown Honolulu, Hawaii. It is the state's designated level II trauma center, and approximately 40 patients with severe TBI are admitted to the 8-bed neuroscience ICU (NSICU) per year (2006–2009). The NSICU mean length of stay for patients with severe TBI is 18 days with a mortality of 28%, average age of 36 years (ranging from 14–69 years), and 95% of patients are male.[10] National statistics differ from these figures, reporting an incidence of TBI of 66% men and 23% women.[1]

As a primary stroke facility and Joint Commission–certified stroke center, an average of 500 patients with stroke diagnosis are admitted per year, with the NSICU admitting an average of 100 patients per year. About 75% of these patients have ischemic disease and 25% of patients have hemorrhagic stroke.[11]

Knowledge and problem triggers underscored the need for an evidence-based treatment protocol to manage fever in the NSICU. While establishing a TBI database for the NSICU, a high incidence and prolonged temperature increase was noted. The database and electronic medical record audits also revealed trends of fever under treatment and inadequate documentation. In the absence of a temperature management protocol, the current practice in the NSICU provided the nurse with a standing order for Tylenol to treat temperature greater than 38.6°C (101.5°F). Adjusting the room thermostat, ice packs, and the use of a circulating fan were noted interventions used by nurses. The use of cooling blankets was infrequent. Current literature confirmed that the issues experienced related to temperature management are not unique to this NSICU.

Forming a Team

A team consisting of 7 neurocritical nurses, a neuroscience clinical nurse specialist (CNS), 2 neuroscience research nurses, and a PhD nurse research mentor met for a total of 12 2-hour meetings during a period of 8 months. The team reviewed and synthesized relevant articles, decided on recommendations for best practices, and developed a written EBP guideline.

Assemble, Critique, and Synthesize Literature

A medical librarian was consulted to assist with assembling the literature. Key words used for the literature search were traumatic brain injury, nursing management, hyperthermia, fever, temperature management, normothermia, and shivering using CINAHL, Medline, PubMed, and the Cochrane databases, with a focus on the past 10 years.

A total of 42 relevant studies were assembled and critiqued using Mosby levels of evidence (**Table 1**).[12] To facilitate literature synthesis, information was organized into a matrix that proved valuable as a quick reference during development of the EBP guideline. Articles were categorized and assigned to a team member to read, critique, and summarize. Categories included scope of the problem, fever definitions, environmental cooling, pharmacologic treatment of fever, ice saline, surface cooling, intravascular cooling, shivering, outcomes, and timing of fever treatment. Each study was critiqued by 2 team members and then discussed as a group to ensure accuracy of grading the evidence. The recurring theme encountered in the literature review validated the need to promote normothermia and nursing management of increased temperature in the neurocritical care patient.

High incidence of fever

The high incidence of fever and secondary injury that results from fever in the neurocritical care patient population is well documented in the literature. Albrecht and

Table 1 Level of evidence	
Number of Articles	**Level of Evidence**
1	Level I: meta-analysis
9	Level II: randomized controlled trial
5	Level III: controlled trial, no randomization
7	Level IV: case control or cohort study, longitudinal studies
5	Level V: correlation study
11	Level VI: descriptive studies
0	Level VII: authority opinion or expert committee reports
4	Reviews: other

From Melnyk B. A focus on adult acute and critical care. Worldviews Evid Based Nurs 2004;1(3):194–7; with permission.

colleagues[13] (1998) reported that fever occurred in 68% of patients with TBI within 72 hours of hospitalization. In a retrospective study of 846 patients with TBI, Jiang and colleagues[14] (2002) reported a 67.5% incidence of fever (>37°C) in the first 48 hours of hospitalization, with a fever greater than 39°C occurring in 25% of the patients. In a retrospective analysis of 110 patients admitted within 24 hours of stroke, fever, and sub-febrility (temperatures 37.5–38°C) were associated with more severe symptoms.[15,16]

Nursing management

Nursing interventions to manage fever are often delayed, and consensus definitions of normothermia, fever, and the temperature at which to initiate protocols varied be-tween institutions, regions, and personal clinical decision making.[17] In a retrospective chart review of 108 neurocritical care patients, only 31% of patients with fever received any documented intervention and delay in implementing a treatment protocol occurred in 58% of patients.[18] A questionnaire mailed to nurses working in neurocrit-ical care units showed that fewer than 20% have a fever management protocol in place for neurologic patients, variations in temperature ranges to start treatment were 37 to 40°C, and choice of pharmacologic therapy was inconsistent. Common findings for treatment across studies are the use of acetaminophen every 4 hours, ice packs, water cooling blankets, and tepid bathing.[19]

Normothermia recommended

Current strategies to improve neurologic outcomes following TBI are multidisciplinary and include the application of the Guidelines for the Management of Severe Traumatic Brain Injury.[20] TBI guidelines cite maintenance of normothermia as the minimum stan-dard of care and recommend mild to moderate hypothermia for neuroprotection and improved patient outcomes.[20] In addition, ischemic stroke guidelines by the American Heart Association state that fever should be treated pharmacologically and with cool-ing measures such as cooling blankets and cooling devices.[21]

Sufficient evidence

The literature clearly supported the necessity to treat fever and maintain normo-thermia. However, there is no definitive research for the steps to achieve normo-thermia in this population. Findings across studies supported the clinical relevance and need for the development of temperature management guidelines for the neuro-critical care patient population.[14–21] A retrospective chart audit of 81 patients with severe TBI in the NSICU at our facility revealed an average daily maximum tempera-ture of 37.6°C, and only 3% of temperature greater than 37.0°C (n = 4247) were noted to have a documented fever reduction intervention (**Table 2**).

IMPLEMENTATION STRATEGIES
Development of the EBP Guideline

There is no clear definition for fever in the literature so defining normothermia and fever was a challenge. A literature summary for fever control and its outcome by Aiyagari and Diringer[5] (2007) provided a range for fever definition between 37°C and 38.5°C. Hoedemaekers and colleagues[22] (2007) defined normothermia at 37.0°C in their tem-perature management study. Diringer[23] (2004) defined fever at greater than 38.0°C when conducting a studying to determine effectiveness of a catheter-based system in reducing increased temperature. After much discussion, the team defined the normothermia threshold at 37.0°C and concluded that it was a valid starting point for a preventive phase of fever management.

Before this project, temperature readings were measured every 4 hours with a tym-panic thermometer or sporadically with a continuous brain temperature/intracranial

Table 2
Preguideline and postguideline data

	Before Guideline (2006–2009) n = 4247[a]	After Guideline (2011) n = 4590[a]	After Guideline (2013) n = 300[b]
Age (y)	44 ± 18	55 ± 17	47
Male gender (%)	79	43	66
Diagnosis	100% TBI	10% TBI 10% ischemic stroke 22% ICH 55% SAH	16% TBI 25% ischemic stroke 25% ICH 33% SAH
Admission temperature (°C)	36.3 ± 1	36.4 ± 1	36.5
Admission GCS	6 ± 2	11 ± 6	10
Discharge GCS	14 ± 2	14 ± 2	—
ICU LOS (d)	18 ± 11	13 ± 7	—
Mortality (%)	25	24	—
Average daily maximum temperature (°C)	37.6	37.8	37.9
T ≥37.0°C (%)	40	69	—
T ≥37.0°C (% treated[c])	3	9.4	—
T ≥37.5°C (% treated[d])	10	15.5	30
Guideline compliance (%)	—	9.4	30
Average temperature nursing treated (°C)	37.8	37.8	38.3
Average temperature nursing did not treat (°C)	37.5	37.6	38.0

Abbreviations: GCS, Glasgow Coma Score; ICH, intracranial hemorrhage; LOS, length of stay; SAH, subarachnoid hemorrhage; T, temperature.
  [a] n = temperature episode ≥37.0°C.
  [b] n = temperature episode ≥37.5°C.
  [c] Initial normothermia definition and threshold T ≥37.0°C.
  [d] Revised normothermia definition and threshold T ≥37.5°C.

pressure monitor. Foley catheters with continuous temperature sensors were made available to our facility as this project evolved. This equipment allowed continuous temperature measurement, which is most suitable for monitoring trends.

The efficacy of pharmacologic interventions alone for fever management is inconclusive,[5] but a retrospective review of temperature interventions in the NSICU suggested that acetaminophen (Tylenol) in combination with external measures, such as surface cooling, cool cloth bath, and reducing the room temperature, may be more effective than acetaminophen (Tylenol) alone (**Fig. 1**). This finding is consistent with an experimental study conducted by Price and colleagues[24] (2003) examining cooling methods for critically ill patients with cerebral insults. Despite the small sample size of 67 patients, the study suggests that acetaminophen in combination with evaporative cooling reduces body core temperature in adult, ventilated patients. The same study discounted the effectiveness of circulating fans.

The use of the Blanketrol III cooling blanket was supported by a prospective, randomized controlled trial, evaluating efficacy and safety of 5 different cooling methods for induction and maintenance of hypothermia and normothermia in critically ill patients.[22] The study results showed that temperature decreased faster in patients

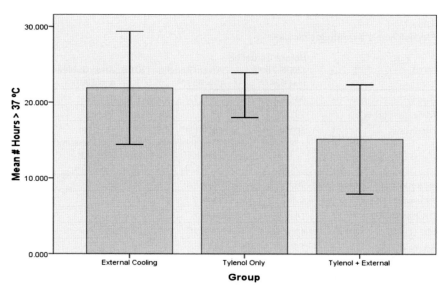

Error Bars: +/- 2 SE

Fig. 1. Temperature interventions in the NSICU. SE, standard error.

cooled with water-circulating blankets, gel-coated cooling pads, and intravascular cooling devices compared with air-circulating cooling devices and conventional methods. Conventional cooling consisted of rapid infusion of cooled intravenous (IV) solution followed by surface cooling using icepacks.

The resulting EBP guideline, entitled *Normothermia for NeuroProtection*, outlines 3 phases of increased temperature with recommended interventions consisting of environmental and evaporative therapies, pharmacologic interventions, surface cooling, and intravascular cooling. The preventive phase (temperature [T] >37°C) primarily consists of environmental, evaporative, and pharmacologic interventions. The therapeutic phase (T>38°C–38.6°C) adds surface cooling with the Blanketrol III cooling vest and blanket. The refractory phase (T>38.6°C) expands the cooling blanket arsenal and includes a cooling head wrap and considerations for intravascular cooling (**Table 3**).

Impact of Shivering

Shivering can occur at normothermic or even hyperthermic stages of temperature because of increases in the hypothalamic thermoregulator set point (fever) and leads to an increasing threshold zone and rewarming.[25] Shivering dramatically increases the amount of heat transfer required to maintain normothermia, and may be associated with adverse effects on level of consciousness, defeat the cooling process, eliminate the potential benefits of therapeutic normothermia, and in extreme cases may be more detrimental than the fever.[26]

In addition to the normothermia guideline, a practice standard to address shivering was also constructed from existing literature recommendations (**Table 4**).[27–33] The Bedside Shivering Assessment Scale (BSAS), a clinical tool that measures severity of shivering, is the basis for the EBP shivering guideline.[28] Evidence-based recommendations for treatment of shivering include pharmacologic and therapeutic interventions, such as counterwarming. Efforts should be focused on avoiding shivering and halting it as soon as it starts; therefore, early recognition, prevention, and treatment are imperative to maximize normothermia interventions.

Table 3
Normothermia for NeuroProtection: NSICU guideline

Preventive Phase Temperature >37.0°C	Therapeutic Phase Temperature >38°C–38.6°C	Refractory Phase Temperature >38.6°C
Environment + pharmacologic therapies	Surface therapies	Core focused therapies
1. Cool room	Institute interventions 1, 2, and 3 listed for the preventive phase	Institute interventions 1, 2, 3, and 4 then:
• Adjust thermostat dial to cool	4. Surface cooling: Blanketrol III blanket and vest	5. Add Blanketrol III head wrap
• Fan not recommended	• Apply blanket on top of patient, set target temperature to 37°C	6. Consider cooled NG instilled fluids
2. Administer Tylenol per MD order		7. Consider cooled IV fluids
• 650 mg q 4 h (recommended)	• Apply vest to patient	8. Suggest Coolgard intravascular cooling for normothermia
• Do not exceed 3900 mg/d	• Set temperature gradient to 20°C with smart mode	Target temperature = 37°C
3. Cool cloth bath (evaporative cooling)	• Assess skin q 4	Points to remember:
• Remove clothing	Points to remember:	• Monitor for S/S of infection
• Use cool tap water to wash all skin surfaces	• Monitor for S/S of infection	• Monitor skin integrity
• Pad dry to prevent shivering	• Monitor skin integrity	• Institute shivering management guidelines
• Place cool cloth on forehead; replace when it becomes warm	• Institute shivering management guidelines	
Combination therapies may be more effective (eg, cool cloth bath and Tylenol)		
Points to remember:		
• Baseline CBC with differential		
• Institute shivering management guidelines		

Abbreviations: CBC, complete blood count; MD, Doctor of Medicine; NG, nasogastric; Q, every; S/S, signs & symptoms.

Educational Strategies and Marketing

A month-long campaign, launched in January 2010, introduced the *Normothermia for NeuroProtection* and *Shivering Management* guidelines to the NSICU nursing staff. The campaign was evident on entrance into the NSICU because nurses were greeted with icicles, snowflakes, and large blue campaign buttons hanging from the ceiling. Inscribed on the button is the campaign theme, "It's Hot to be COOL 37°C" (**Fig. 2**). The event was highlighted with hospital-wide presentations at monthly nursing grand rounds, unit based registered nurse (RN) and advanced practice RN (APRN) in-services, and inclusion of content into the annual competency fair. Laminated copies of the guidelines were placed in each patient room, providing easy access.

A contest with incentives was established to encourage staff to adhere to the guideline and draw attention to the campaign. Staff nurses received a point each time a temperature reduction intervention was initiated as per the guideline. The neuro-CNS kept a cumulative point tally for a period of 4 weeks, which culminated with 2 nurses with

Table 4
Shivering management: NSICU guideline

	0 = Absent	1 = Mild	2 = Moderate	3 = Severe
	Absence of shivering on neck or pectoral muscles	Localized to the neck and/or thorax. May be present only on palpation	Involvement of the UE ± neck or pectoralis muscles	Generalized whole-body involvement
	Goal = BSAS ≤1 Every hour: palpate masseter, pectoralis, deltoids, and quadriceps muscles for shivering. Watch for fine quivering in electrocardiogram, or BIS tracing			
Interventions[a]	Optimize sedation and analgesia	Acetaminophen Buspar + meperidine Magnesium IV gtt	Buspar + meperidine Magnesium IV continuous Dexmedetomidine Fentanyl	Must be on ventilator: Propofol Paralytics
Counterwarming	—	Place warm socks or blanket on hands and feet	Place warm socks or blanket on hands and feet	Consider Bair Hugger at 40–43°C

Buspirone (Buspar; pharmacologically reduces the shiver threshold; best if given with Demerol). Suggested dosing:
- Initial dose of 30 mg feeding tube then, 15–20 mg q 8
- Usual dose required is 20–30 mg/d in 2–3 divided doses; maximum dose 60 mg/d

Meperidine (Demerol; pharmacologically reduces the shiver threshold; synergistic with Buspar). Suggested dosing:
- 12.5–50 mg intravenously 3–4 times a day or as a continuous infusion up to 24 h
- if CR <2 and UOP >30 mL/h, reduce dose

Dexmedetomidine (Precedex; reduces both the vasoconstriction and shivering thresholds). Suggested dosing:
- 0.2–1.5 μg/kg/h IV. Hold for HR <50 bpm or SBP <90 mm Hg

Propofol (Diprivan; to provide shiver suppression and continuous sedation). Suggested dosing:
- 20 μg/kg/min IV, titrate by 5 μg/kg/min as needed (not to exceed 50 μg/kg/min)

Vecuronium (Nocuron); only after adequate sedation is achieved; BIS ≤60). Suggested dosing:
- 0.1 mg/kg (up to 10 mg) IVP intermittent boluses prn shivering

Magnesium IV (vasodilation; improves efficacy of cooling and increases patient comfort; maintain high normal levels). Suggested dosing:
- 12 g in 250 mL NS; continuous infusion at 0.5–1.0 g/h (10 mL/h); titrate to maintain a serum magnesium level of 3–4 mg/dL
- Monitor levels

[a] Requires MD order.

Abbreviations: BIS, bispectral index; bpm, beats per minute; BSAS, Bedside Shivering Assessment Scale; CR, creatinine; gtt, drip; HR, heart rate; IVP, IV push; NS, normal saline; prn, as needed; SBP, systolic blood pressure; UE, upper extremities; UOP, urine output.

Data from Refs.[27–33]

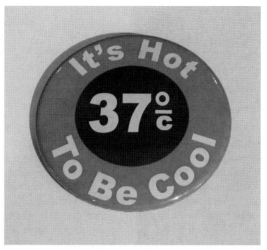

Fig. 2. Normothermia for NeuroProtection and Shivering Management campaign button.

the most points receiving a first prize Apple Store gift card and second prize with a spa gift certificate. The contest produced a tie with 2 first-place winners who were very engaged and set the tone for healthy competition. All the contest winners proved to be enthusiastic supporters of the new practice change. Feedback on the guideline was solicited at this time.

A hallmark of the normothermia guideline is the use of the Blanketrol III, a surface cooling device. Ongoing in-services about the use of the machine were provided on the unit and one-on-one training occurred at the bedside in the rooms of patients requiring cooling measures. Collaboration with the central supply department to ensure availability of supplies was essential to success. The increased use of the Blanketrol III required purchasing of additional machines and upgrades for older models. Introduction of expanded uses of surface cooling included use of a cooling vest and head wrap to supplement the traditional body blanket.

EVALUATION

The new practice changes created initial excitement but maintaining the momentum proved challenging. Many applauded the 3-phase intervention model, which places emphasis on prevention and early intervention when the patient's temperature begins to trend up. The staff recognized the impact of early treatment and acknowledged that it was less laborious to prevent a fever spike than to bring down a high fever. The following are examples of the initial feedback received from staff: "Guidelines are great…the emphasis to treat temperatures greater than 37°C is smart, then we avoid having to chase high fevers such as 38–40°C." "I love the whole concept of the preventive phase…when I treat temps as soon as they're greater than 37°C, the treatments are effective (Tylenol, cool wash cloths under armpits or on head) and I don't even have to do anything more physical such as (place a Blanketrol III)." "It great!!! Sometimes we work harder than we really need to… why wait to have to turn a heavy patient and place the Blanketrol III when we can give Tylenol or a cool bath as soon as we see the temp rising? Thanks again!"

Monitoring Practice Change

An anonymous survey to identify facilitators and barriers to guideline adherence was administered to 28 eligible NSICU nurses. To be eligible, RNs must have worked in the

NSICU as a staff nurse during the entire implementation period of the EBP guidelines (normothermia and shivering), must consent to participate, and be willing to speak up regarding their perceptions on use of the EBP guidelines. Twenty-seven surveys were returned for analysis. **Box 1** list the 5 questions included in the staff nurse survey, which produced responses with common themes. The facilitators and barriers to guideline implementation are summarized in **Box 2**.

Nursing Compliance

To determine the impact of the practice change, it was important to measure nursing compliance with the temperature management guideline. A retrospective chart audit 10 months after guideline implementation identified temperature points greater than 37.0°C. Of the 4590 temperatures taken, there was a daily average maximum temperature of 37.8°C. Compared with 3% compliance with 4247 temperatures taken at the preintervention data collection point, 9.4% of temperature increases greater than or equal to 37.0°C were treated with fever reduction interventions (see **Table 2**). Continued monitoring 18 months after guideline implementation revealed an average daily maximum temperature of 37.9°C and 30% compliance with the guideline for temperatures greater than or equal to 37.5°C. This is an improvement from the 10% before the guideline, and the 15.5% after the guideline in 2011 when evaluating compliance with treating temperature greater than or equal to 37.5°C. The difference in the patient sampling was attributed to the literature supporting temperature management for all patients with neurologic injury and especially patients with a stroke diagnosis.

LESSONS LEARNED
What Worked?

Introduction of a new practice and sustaining the change is challenging and ongoing. Numerous factors contribute to the success of the implementation of normothermia and shivering guidelines in the NSICU. Credit is given to the team involved in the project, especially the staff nurses engaged at the bedside and recognizing the importance of being proactive in the management of increased temperature.

The It's Hot to be Cool campaign was a successful vehicle to launch the new practice recommendations. It created attention, excitement, and a source of discussion during the first few weeks. The campaign buttons that were distributed left a lasting impression, because name tags and back packs were decorated with them weeks thereafter. The campaign was primarily targeted for the NSICU, but presenting the project at monthly nursing grand rounds provided hospital-wide exposure and produced interest from other departments.

Box 1
Staff RN survey

Thoughts on implementing the temperature management EBP guideline

Your initial date of hire at the NSICU, Queen's Medical Center: (month, year)

1. When you hear the words, temperature management, what comes to mind?
2. When you hear the words, evidence-based practice guideline, what comes to mind?
3. Tell me about those processes that have facilitated the implementation of the temperature management guideline.
4. Tell me about those processes that have created barriers to guideline implementation.
5. When implementing an EBP guideline, what do you think is most important?

| Box 2 |
| Summary of barriers and facilitators to guidelines |

What created barriers to guideline implementation?

- Old habits are hard to break
- Some staff with negative opinion of guidelines
- Increased nurse workload
- Increased patient acuity
- Equipment malfunction and unavailable
- Inadequate supplies
- Lack of order sets
- MD (Doctor of Medicine) orders not consistent with guideline
- Lack of support and reinforcement from MD

What facilitated implementation of guideline?

- Printed accessible guideline algorithm
- Functional equipment
- Continuous bladder temperature monitor
- MD support
- Education, competency inclusion
- Nurse manager and education council support
- Accessible guideline algorithm
- Motivating staff
- Physician support

A hospital-wide team was concurrently in the process of developing hypothermia after cardiac arrest (HACA) guidelines that included cooling and shivering management. Although the focus of HACA is hypothermia, the aggressive cooling outlined in the refractory phase of the NSICU normothermia guideline outlines use of the Coolgard intravascular device and was used in the HACA protocol as a primary intervention. A modified version of NSCIU's shivering guideline was adopted by the team.

Designing simple 1-page algorithms accessible in all patient rooms proved helpful in facilitating implementation of the guidelines. The tiered phases of temperature intervention received positive feedback from the nursing staff. The nurse is given a starting point that supports autonomy in selecting interventions appropriate for the temperature range. It encourages nurses to consider combinations of interventions focused on prevention, which is less tedious than having to reduce a highly increased temperature.

The introduction of temperature-sensing urinary catheters in the critical care units also proved timely and advantageous to our guideline launching. The availability of continuous temperature readings facilitated surveillance of escalating trends and helped trigger early intervention. In addition, the newly purchased Blanketrol III hypothermia machines provided a compatible connection to the urinary catheter.

What Were the Challenges?

The process of implementing new practice change presented new challenges for the NSICU staff. One challenge identified by staff as being evident early after implementation was the increase in workload attributed to early intervention, but necessary for the maintenance of normothermia and the required escalating treatments. Supported by the NSICU nurse manager and a patient acuity system, adjustment to staffing assignments were made to accommodate the additional workload.

Controlling shivering contributes significantly to patient acuity and created frustration among staff who verbalized shivering as a significant barrier to guideline implementation. In addition, varying physician approaches for shivering prevention and treatment were often viewed by nurses as inconsistent and contrary to the shivering guideline, which may have discouraged nurses from aggressive temperature intervention. There are several nurse-driven interventions in the guideline that combat shivering; however, many are pharmacologic and require a physician order.

The creation of order sets to initiate normothermia and shivering management were requested by staff. However, varying patient conditions and differences in practice preferences among the neurointensivists in the NSICU hindered the use of standard order sets. Staff feedback included, "Different doctors have different treatment modalities and don't follow guidelines/protocols" and "(There are) inconsistent orders because we have three different MDs."

Operational concerns with the use of the Blanketrol III hypothermia machine were initial contributors to workflow challenges. To accommodate workflow, some thought and planning was required for placement of the machine and the hose attachments in an already crowded room. The use of the vest and head wrap was considered cumbersome by the staff and the different modes of operation complex and difficult to set up, which became problematic when nurses, in an effort to speed up cooling, would attempt to manually adjust the blanket temperature, causing a drastic reduction and often triggering early shivering. To address these issues, company representatives were consulted and provided additional in-services for the staff. These issues are now mostly resolved.

Recommendations

The guideline does not fit all patients, especially those who are awake and not sedated. The use of the hypothermia blanket recommended in the therapeutic phase may be particularly counterproductive in this patient group because of shivering. The nurse must consider the distress and discomfort this would cause the patient. Interventions listed in the preventive phase may be more appropriate and are less likely to cause shivering.

Note the amendment of the normothermia threshold from 37.0°C to 37.5°C. The expectation to begin temperature reduction interventions at 37.0°C was not practical and premature treatment may mask initial signs of infections. Reexamination of the existing literature revealed that a large number of studies used 37.5°C as the fever threshold. Thus, we have now revised our normothermia guideline.

Although cost is not readily recognized at the bedside, the impact on patient hospitalization must be acknowledged. Once initiated, normothermia management is likely to continue for several days or more. There is an additional nursing resource requirement caused by increased patient acuity. There is also a need for additional equipment and supplies for pharmacologic use for both normothermia management and shivering prevention. However, these additional costs may be offset by earlier discharge from the NSICU and/or hospital, less loss of disability, and improved long-term function. It would be beneficial to include a cost-benefit analysis in future projects.

SUMMARY

Fever is a significant contributor to secondary brain insult and management is a challenge for the neurocritical care team. The absence of standardized guidelines likely contributes to poor surveillance and undertreatment of increased temperature. A need for practice change was identified and this EBP project was initiated to compile sufficient evidence to develop, implement, and evaluate a treatment guideline to manage fever and maintain normothermia in the neurocritical care population. Sustaining and monitoring the use of the normothermia and shivering management guidelines are ongoing processes. The improvement in guideline compliance is encouraging and the goal is to continue to monitor performance through quality improvement audits. Ongoing education, inclusion in NSICU staff annual competency, and staff update on compliance performance is essential to maintain and sustain the practice change achieved through this project.

ACKNOWLEDGMENTS

The authors would like to acknowledge the following individuals for their support of this project. EBP team: Susan Asai, RN; Dan Choe, RN; Jodie Kaalekahi, RN; Kim Nguyen, RN; Lyle Oshita, RN; Sandra Talavera, RN; Cherylee Chang, MD, Director, Neuroscience Institute; Johnna DeCastillo; Cindy Kamikawa, RN, CNO, The Queen's Medical Center; Kawehi Kauhola, RN, Manager, Neuroscience ICU; Matthew Koenig, MD; Renee Latimer, RN, Director, Queen Emma Nursing Institute; Dongmei Li, MS, PhD; Joseph Mobley Jr, PhD; Kazuma Nakagawa, MD; Dalnam Park; Neuroscience ICU staff.

REFERENCES

1. Langlois JA, Rutland-Brown W, Thomas KE. Traumatic brain injury in the United States: emergency department visits, hospitalizations, and deaths. Atlanta (GA): Centers for Disease Control and Prevention, National Center for Injury Prevention and Control; 2006.
2. Roger VL, Go AS, Lloyd-Jones DM, et al. Heart disease and stroke statistics—2012 update: a report from the American Heart Association. Circulation 2012; 125:e2–220.
3. Heidenreich PA, Trogdon JG, Khavjou OA, et al. Forecasting the future of cardiovascular disease in the United States: a policy statement from the American Heart Association. Circulation 2011;123:933–44.
4. Balabis J, Pubotsky A, Baker KK, et al. The burden of cardiovascular disease in Hawaii 2007. Honolulu (HI): Hawaii State Department of Health; 2007.
5. Aiyagari V, Diringer MN. Fever control and its impact on outcomes: what is the evidence? J Neurol Sci 2007;261:39–46.
6. Fritz HG, Bauer R. Secondary injuries in brain trauma: effects of hypothermia. J Neurosurg Anesthesiol 2004;16:43–52.
7. Greer DM, Funk SE, Reaven NL, et al. Impact of fever on outcome in patients with stroke and neurologic injury: a comprehensive meta-analysis. Stroke 2008;39: 3029–35.
8. Diringer MN, Reaven MA, Funk SE, et al. Elevated body temperature independently contributes to increased length of stay in neurologic intensive care unit patients. Crit Care Med 2004;32:1489–95.
9. Titler MG, Kleiber C, Rakel B, et al. The Iowa Model of evidence-based practice to promote quality care. Crit Care Nurs Clin North Am 2001;13:497–509.

10. The Queen's Medical Center, Trauma Database. Traumatic Brain Injury Quality Improvement Program: TBI-trac™, 2006–2009.

11. The Queen's Medical Center, Neuroscience Institute, Stroke Database, 2009.

12. Melnyk BM. A focus on adult acute and critical care. Worldviews Evid Based Nurs 2004;1(3):194–7 Modified from Guyatt & Rennie (2002), Harris et al. (2001).

13. Albrecht RF 2nd, Wass CT, Lanier WL. Occurrence of potentially detrimental temperature alterations in hospitalized patients at risk for brain injury. Mayo Clin Proc 1998;73:629–35.

14. Jiang JY, Gao GY, Li WP, et al. Early indicators of prognosis in 846 cases of severe traumatic brain injury. J Neurotrauma 2002;19:869–74.

15. Hindfelt B. The prognostic significance of subfebrility and fever in ischemic cerebral infarction. Acta Neurol Scand 1976;53:72–9.

16. Ginsberg MD, Busto R. Combating hyperthermia in acute stroke: a significant clinical concern. Stroke 1998;29:529–34.

17. Thompson HJ, Kirkness CJ, Mitchell PH. Intensive care unit management of fever following traumatic brain injury. Intensive Crit Care Nurs 2007;23:91–6.

18. Thompson HJ, Kirkness CJ, Mitchell PH, et al. Fever management practices of neuroscience nurses: national and regional perspectives. J Neurosci Nurs 2007;39:151–62.

19. Thompson HJ, Kirkness CJ, Mitchell PH, et al. Fever management practices of neuroscience nurses, part II: nurse, patients, and barriers. J Neurosci Nurs 2007;39:196–201.

20. Brain Trauma Foundation, American Association of Neurological Surgeons, Congress of Neurological Surgeons, et al. Guidelines for the management of severe traumatic brain injury. XV. Steroids. J Neurotrauma 2007;24(Suppl 1):S91–5.

21. Adams HP Jr, del Zoppo G, Alberts MJ, et al. Guidelines for the early management of adults with ischemic stroke: a guideline from the American Heart Association/American Stroke Association Stroke Council, Clinical Cardiology Council, Cardiovascular Radiology and Intervention Council, and the Atherosclerotic Peripheral Vascular Disease and Quality of Care Outcomes in Research Interdisciplinary Working Groups: the American Academy of Neurology affirms the value of this guideline as an educational tool for neurologists. Stroke 2007;38: 1655–711.

22. Hoedemaekers CW, Ezzahti M, Gerritsen A, et al. Comparison of cooling methods to induce and maintain normo- and hypothermia in intensive care patients: a prospective intervention study. Crit Care 2007;1:R91.

23. Diringer MN. Treatment of fever in the neurologic intensive care unit with a catheter-based heat exchange system. Crit Care Med 2004;32:559–64.

24. Price T, McGloin S, Izzard J, et al. Cooling strategies for patients with severe cerebral insult in ICU (Part 2). Nurs Crit Care 2003;8:37–45.

25. Holtzclaw BJ. Shivering in acutely ill vulnerable populations. AACN Clin Issues 2004;15:267–79.

26. Badjatia NJ, Kowalski RG, Schimidt JM, et al. Predictors and clinical implications of shivering during therapeutic normothermia. Neurocrit Care 2007;6:186–91.

27. Badjatia N, Strongilis E, Prescutti M, et al. Metabolic benefits of surface counter warming during therapeutic temperature modulation. Crit Care Med 2009;37:1–5.

28. Badjatia NJ, Strongilis E, Gordon E, et al. Metabolic impact of shivering during therapeutic temperature modulation. Stroke 2008;39:3242–7.

29. Choi H, Ko S, Presciutti M, et al. Prevention of shivering during therapeutic temperature modulation: the Columbia Anti-Shivering Protocol. Neurocrit Care 2011; 14:389–94.

30. Doufas A, Wadhwa A, Lin C, et al. Neither arm nor face warming reduces the shivering threshold in unanesthetized humans. Stroke 2003;34:1736–40.
31. Kizilirmak S, Karakas S, Akca O, et al. Magnesium sulfate stops post anesthetic shivering. Ann N Y Acad Sci 1997;813:799–806.
32. Mokhtarani M, Mahgoub A, Morioka N, et al. Buspirone and meperidine synergistically reduce the shivering threshold. Anesth Analg 2001;93:1233–9.
33. Talke P, Tayefeh S, Sessler D, et al. Dexmedetomidine does not alter the sweating threshold, but comparably and linearly decreases the vasoconstriction and shivering thresholds. Anesthesiology 1997;87:835–41.

Improving Pain Management in Orthopedic Surgical Patients with Opioid Tolerance

Kathleen Doi, APRN, MS, CNS[a],*, Rosanne Shimoda, RN[b],
Gregory Gibbons, BSN, CCRN, CPAN, CAPA[c]

KEYWORDS

- Pain management • Orthopedic • Opioid tolerance • Joint replacement

KEY POINTS

- The surgical intervention for osteoarthritis of aging joints is joint replacement surgery.
- Patients undergoing total hip and knee replacements usually endure chronic pain before their surgeries and are seeking surgical relief in record numbers.
- The trigger for an evidence-based practice project on improving pain management occurred when the Pain Service and Nursing Departments noted the difficulties experienced by orthopedic surgical patients with opioid tolerance.
- The purpose of this project was to identify strategies and develop best practices for pain management in this surgical joint replacement patient population.

INTRODUCTION

The combination of an aging baby boomer population, implementation of health care reform, and increased prevalence of opioid use could be considered a perfect storm, creating major challenges to health care delivery today. As the population ages, growing numbers of patients have osteoarthritis. Fifty million Americans have some form of arthritis or other rheumatic condition. That number is expected to climb to 67 million, an increase of 25%, by the year 2030.[1] These patients frequently use opioids for chronic pain management of osteoarthritis and often acquire mechanisms of tolerance and dependence.[2]

Disclosures: None.
[a] Pain Service, Kaiser Moanalua Medical Center, 3288 Moanalua Road, Honolulu, HI 96819, USA; [b] Preoperative Evaluation and Education Center, Kaiser Moanalua Medical Center, 3288 Moanalua Road, Honolulu, HI 96819, USA; [c] Post Anesthesia Care Unit, Kaiser Moanalua Medical Center, 3288 Moanalua Road, Honolulu, HI 96819, USA
* Corresponding author.
E-mail address: kathleen.doi@kp.org

Nurs Clin N Am 49 (2014) 415–429
http://dx.doi.org/10.1016/j.cnur.2014.05.015
0029-6465/14/$ – see front matter © 2014 Elsevier Inc. All rights reserved.
nursing.theclinics.com

The surgical intervention for osteoarthritis of aging joints is joint replacement surgery. Patients undergoing total hip and knee replacements usually endure chronic pain before their surgeries and are seeking surgical relief in record numbers. It is projected that the increase in demand for joint replacement surgeries will be 174% for primary total hip arthroplasty, 673% increase for total knee arthroplasty, and 137% for total hip revision by the year 2030.[3]

Patients regularly using opioids for pain management before surgery are at risk for increased postoperative pain, greater opioid consumption, and prolonged use of health care resources to manage their pain.[4] Therefore, the purpose of this project was to use an evidence-based practice (EBP) methodology to identify strategies and implement the best practices for pain management in this population of orthopedic surgical joint patients with opioid tolerance.

EVIDENCE-BASED PRACTICE MODEL

The Iowa Model of Evidence-Based Practice to Promote Quality Care provided the framework for this evidence-based nursing project.[5] The Iowa Model starts with the identification of a trigger or problem. If the problem is a priority for the organization, then a team is formed. The composition of the team includes key stakeholders, staff nurses, and other champions of EBP. The next step is finding, critiquing, and synthesizing the evidence. Then, a pilot of practice change occurs, incorporating the evidence that supports the change. Finally, an evaluation of the change process and outcomes that resulted from the practice changes is done.

Triggers

At a 285-bed tertiary medical center in Hawaii, both the Pain Service and Nursing Department noticed a trend of opioid-tolerant surgical patients experiencing poor pain control, delays in rehabilitation, and decreased patient satisfaction. Considerable time and resources were being used to manage their pain. There were also increased referrals to the Pain Service from the Medical/Surgical units and the Postanesthesia Care Unit (PACU) for pain management of opioid-tolerant patients.

Organizational Priority

The increasing changes in health care reimbursement and increasing numbers of the Medicare population have placed a greater emphasis on quality of care and costs. Health care organizations are focused on improvements that maximize opportunities to improve the patient's satisfaction with pain management and decrease hospital utilization costs and length of stay (LOS). This organization takes pride in being the only 5-star–rated Medicare facility within the state, and the focus on improving care for this population was deemed a high priority by the leadership.

Form a Team

The orthopedic surgeon and the Pain Service physician joined forces with nursing services to review the current process of care. Several staff nurses who were interested in improving the care for opioid-tolerant patients and in the EBP process volunteered to join the team. The team was formed and included both clinic and hospital nursing staff. Nursing management strongly supported this project. The team felt the changes would affect several services, and members were selected to represent these areas. The team membership included staff from the Orthopedic Clinic, Perioperative Evaluation and Education Center (PEEC), PACU, and the Medical/Surgical unit in which most of the orthopedic patients received postoperative care.

Physician leadership in both Orthopedics and Pain Service participated in the EBP changes and supported the team. The physician participation was evident as they utilized and implemented the practice changes.

EVIDENCE FOR PRACTICE IMPROVEMENT
Literature Search

A literature search was conducted using PubMed, CINAHL, and OVID and yielded 63 citations that provided evidence for practice strategies and changes. Search terms included *arthroplasty, preemptive medication, opioid, preoperative assessment, orthopedic, multimodal analgesia*, and *total knee and hip replacement*. The citations were critiqued by the EBP team members over the course of several months. The levels of evidence for the literature search were tabulated using Mosby's level of evidence scale (**Fig. 1**).

Literature Synthesis

A summary of findings from the literature recommended: (1) preoperative patient evaluation and planning,[6,7] (2) preemptive medication use and incorporation of multimodal pain strategies,[8] (3) enhanced communication approaches within and between provider disciplines,[9] (4) patient education about pain management and beneficial mutual goal setting between patients and caregivers,[10] and (5) staff education to enhance implementation of pain interventions.[11]

The following practice changes were incorporated into the guideline.

- Early and improved identification of opioid-tolerant patients before surgery with development and use of a pain screening tool and adoption of systematic interventions to improve pain management
  - Incorporation of Pain Service physician recommendations in all perioperative phases, continuation of analgesics used preoperatively to avoid analgesic gaps in patient care, and earlier initiation of patient-controlled analgesia (PCA)
- Implementation of a new internal process to enhance communication
  - Notification system via the electronic medical record (EMR), visual reminders of opioid-tolerant patients, and improved handoffs in patient transfers of care
- Enhanced patient and family education instructions concerning pain management
  - Earlier preoperative education about pain management, setting mutual pain goals, and consistent patient instructions through all phases of the surgical experience

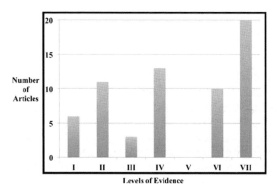

Fig. 1. Number and levels of evidence.

- Improved competency in pain management via staff education
  - Timely medication interventions to avoid pain escalation and prolonged episodes of pain
  - Increased collaboration with physicians and use of multimodal pain adjuncts

Baseline Data

Retrospective chart reviews were done on 20 patients who had undergone joint replacement surgery to gain an understanding of the patients' courses of care. Data collected included patient demographics, preoperative and postoperative pain medication (both opioid and nonopioid), surgical anesthesia, pain scores, and outcome information (**Table 1**). The chart reviews reinforced findings from the literature review and provided the data targeted for change.

Findings included:

- Absence of comprehensive plan of care for pain management in opioid-tolerant patients
- Opportunities to improve pain scores in both the PACU and the Medical/Surgical unit
- Minimal use of multimodal and preemptive analgesics
- Inconsistent timing when administering as-needed pain medications

IMPLEMENTATION STRATEGIES

Evidence from the literature yielded several key interventions to improve pain management for the joint replacement patient population. The decision was made to divide interventions among the phases of care that most surgical patients transition through: preoperative, intraoperative, and postoperative. All of the practice changes that led to guideline development were viewed conceptually as pieces of a puzzle that fit together to achieve the goal of improved patient care (**Fig. 2**).

Preoperative Phase

The preoperative phase included: (1) early identification of opioid-tolerant patients, (2) development of a pain screening tool, (3) creation of a process for referral to Pain Service, (4) inclusion of a multidisciplinary team, and (5) enhanced patient and family education. Although health care providers were aware of the patient's opioid history, information about the quantities taken or duration of use was not well recognized.

"Preexisting pain, chronic pain, low preoperative pain threshold, anxiety (or other psychological distress), age, and type of surgery are the most common variables

Table 1
Baseline data

Patient Demographics	Preoperative	Intraoperative	Postoperative PACU	Postoperative Medical Surgical Unit
Age	Opioids	Anesthesia type	PCA started in PACU	Opioids name, Rx
Sex	Name/dosing	Nerve block	Total time in PACU	Nonopioids name, Rx
Type of surgery	Nonopioids for pain	PCA	Pain scores in PACU	Postoperative complications
Illicit drug use	Preoperative Pain Scores	Epidural		Hospital LOS
Alcohol use				Postoperative pain scores

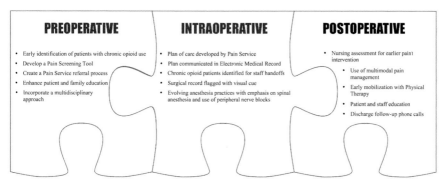

Fig. 2. Phases of Care and Implementation Plan for Opioid-Tolerant Patients.

consistently found to be significant predictors for postoperative pain."[6] Early identification of the opioid-tolerant patient provides an opportunity to engage in realistic goal setting for pain management and allows for enhanced patient education with relevance to the type of analgesia planned for the patient. A pain screening tool was developed to assist in early patient identification (**Fig. 3**). Parameters assessed included: (1) use of opioids; (2) over-the-counter and anxiety medications; (3) illicit substances, including alcohol; and (4) previous orthopedic surgery.

Patients identified as opioid-tolerant were referred to the Pain Service physician who reviewed the EMR and formulated the pain management plan of care (POC) to include recommendations specific to the patient's condition (**Box 1**). The POC was communicated to the surgeon, anesthesiologist, and PEEC staff who provide preoperative education to the patient and family.

Before implementation, interviews with staff revealed that information received from the Pain Service physicians was often difficult to locate in the EMR. Unnecessary time was spent trying to locate the documentation, which resulted in recommendations not being followed. Information technology support assisted with developing an electronic notification system that provided automated communication to all providers involved in the management of pain. Patient education and pain management improved because of a consistent approach and electronic reminders that provided better identification of the opioid-tolerant patient with special needs.

The Pain Service physician frequently incorporated the use of both multimodal and preemptive pain medications when developing the pain management POC. A multimodal approach to pain control involves administration of a combination of multiple analgesics or modalities at various times during the surgical hospitalization.[12] The value of a multimodal approach is that the lowest effective analgesic dose of each drug can be administered resulting in fewer or less-severe adverse effects.[13] Preemptive analgesia, defined as analgesic intervention provided before surgery to prevent or reduce subsequent pain, attempts to prevent the establishment of central sensitization and thereby reduces pain intensity and analgesic requirements.[14]

Intraoperative Phase

The creation of communication tools within the EMR allowed all providers to locate the pain management POC. Staff awareness of the POC also improved communication handoffs during the transfer of patient care. Additionally, the surgical record was flagged with a visual cue that took the form of a laminated sign noting, *Pain Management Patient*. This allowed the preoperative, operating room, anesthesia, and PACU

Surgeon Name: _____

ALL INFORMATION IS CONFIDENTIAL
Place a √ in the box that applies:

1. Do you take any of the following pain medications on a <u>daily</u> basis?

□ NO   Dose   How many tablets/   How long have you
                                  How often?   taken this medication?

□ YES→   □ Fentanyl/Duragesic Patch   _____   _____   _____

             □ Methadone   _____   _____   _____

             □ Morphine SR   _____   _____   _____

             □ Opana ER (oxymorphone)   _____   _____   _____

             □ Oxycontin   _____   _____   _____

             □ Suboxone   _____   _____   _____

2. Do you take any of the following medications <u>as needed</u> for pain?

□ NO   Dose   How many tablets/   How long have you
                                  How often?   taken this medication?

□ YES→   □ Dilaudid (hydromorphone)   _____   _____   _____

             □ Morphine IR   _____   _____   _____

             □ Oxycodone   _____   _____   _____

             □ Percocet/Endocet   _____   _____   _____

             □ Vicodin   _____   _____   _____

             □ Other: _____   _____   _____   _____

3. Do you take any medication to help manage your anxiety?

□ NO   Dose   How many tablets/   How long have you
                                  How often?   taken this medication?

□ YES→ Medication: _____   _____   _____

                        _____   _____   _____

4. Do you take any over-the-counter medications? (Motrin, Tylenol, Ibuprofen, Aspirin, etc.)

□ NO   Dose   How many tablets/   How long have you
                                  How often?   taken this medication?

□ YES→ Medication: _____   _____   _____

                        _____   _____   _____

5. Do you drink alcohol?   **How much do you drink <u>in a week</u>?**

    □ NO→ Did you ever drink alcohol? □ Beer □ Wine □ Liquor _____

    □ YES→   □ Beer □ Wine □ Liquor _____

    □ **History of alcohol use**: how much/how often, when did you stop? _____

6. Do you use "street drugs"?   **How taken (smoke, snort, inject, or swallow)?**

    □ NO→ Did you ever use street drugs? □ Cocaine   □ Crystal Meth

                                       □ Marijuana □ Other: _____

    □ YES→ □ Cocaine □ Crystal Meth   □ Marijuana □ Other: _____

    □ **History of drug use**: how much/how often, when did you stop? _____

7. Have you had joint replacement surgery to the same knee or hip in the past?   □ **NO**   □ **YES**

Fig. 3. Pain Screening Tool.

staff to immediately identify a patient who was opioid-tolerant and implement medication strategies without delay. Strategies included giving preemptive medication or early administration of an oral opioid to achieve optimal pain control and decreasing intraoperative opioid requirements. This also created opportunities to prevent potential analgesic gaps that could occur postoperatively. Evolving anesthesia practices with emphasis on spinal anesthesia and use of peripheral nerve blocks were trends seen in the pain management POC.

Box 1
Example of Pain Service physician plan of care

Patient Name and MR #

RECOMMENDATIONS/PLAN: Recommendations are made with the understanding that the anesthesiologist will provide the appropriate care based on the patient's assessment on the day of surgery

PREOPERATIVE:

- Continue current doses of Opana ER and oxycodone IR
- Lyrica 75 mg po × 1, one to two hours prior to surgery

INTRAOPERATIVE:

- Regional anesthesia per anesthesiologist
- Ketorolac 30 mg IV × 1

POSTOPERATIVE:

- Continue Opana ER 20 mg po q 12 hrs
- Dilaudid IV PCA 0.2 mg per hr (may need 0.3 mg), 0.4 mg q 8 minutes, clinician bolus 1 mg IV q 2 hrs prn severe pain
- Lyrica 25 mg po q 8 hrs
- Ketorolac 30 mg IV q 6 hrs × 48 hrs (if no contraindications)
- Methocarbamol 1000 mg po q 6 hrs prn pain/spasm
- Continuous pulse oximetry

POD #1:

- Discontinue continuous rate on IV PCA
- Increase Opana to 25 mg po q 12 hrs

POD #2:

- Discontinue IV PCA
- Begin oxycodone 10 mg (may need 15 mg) po q 3 hrs prn pain

Postoperative Phase

The postoperative phase included improved nursing assessment for earlier pain intervention, use of multimodal pain management, enhanced communication among providers, improved patient and staff education, and discharge follow-up phone calls.

Pain assessment provides information to make subsequent pain intervention decisions and provide optimal pain relief.[11] Educating nurses about the importance of early pain assessment and appropriate intervention is critical for optimal postoperative care. Assisting patients with setting realistic goals can help them become more active participants in their plan of care and allow them to meet or exceed their expectations of pain management.[15] Using tangible evidence of goal achievement, such as a visible board documenting progress, provides the patient with awareness of improvement. With better pain management, earlier mobilization with physical therapy is possible and can lead to earlier discharge from the hospital.[16]

The timely administration of both pharmacologic and nonpharmacologic pain interventions can provide effective pain management and avoid escalation and continuation of elevated pain levels. Increasing the nurse's knowledge about nerve blocks proved instrumental in learning when supplemental medication would be most helpful. Understanding about the usual duration of the block clarified questions about when to administer additional medications for optimal pain management. Additionally, knowledge gained about the use of both long-acting and short-acting opioids clarified how best to administer them and achieve improved pain management. Use of nonpharmacologic measures, such as cryotherapy, relaxation, guided imagery, and aromatherapy, also provided patients with other alternatives for management of their pain.

Knowledge about the theoretical basis of multimodal strategies for pain management enhanced the nurse's ability and collaboration with physicians in utilizing other pain adjuncts before simply escalating opioids. These adjuncts included the use of muscle relaxants, anti-inflammatory medications, nonsteroidal medications, and acetaminophen-based medications.

The transfer hand off reports between nursing units and within the unit addressed the patient's pain POC. The improved communication and identification of the patient with chronic pain increased staff's knowledge about chronic pain and resulted in caregivers sharing strategies for effective pain management.

Posthospitalization telephone calls with the patients were done to assess and intervene in any continued problems after discharge. The focus was on pain; however, most of the feedback and concerns were about upcoming appointments and very few questions about pain management. The pain questions were mostly about refills, and those with pain concerns were usually referred to the Pain Clinic. The process flow for this project shows the various services involved in the care of the patient and the changes incorporated for improvement in the care of the opioid-tolerant patient (**Fig. 4**). The goal was to provide seamless flow though the continuum of care.

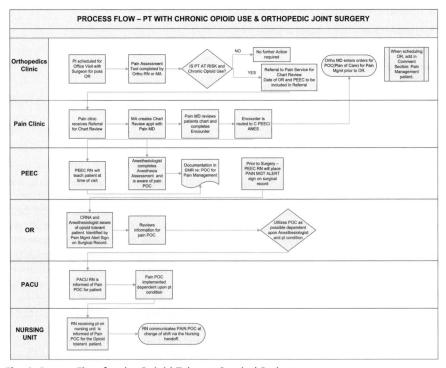

Fig. 4. Process Flow for the Opioid-Tolerant Surgical Patient.

EVALUATION

The implementation of the practice guideline for opioid-tolerant patients had a positive impact on patient satisfaction with pain management and cost savings. To evaluate the results of the practice changes, comparative chart reviews were done for 20 opioid-tolerant patients who did not receive care per the guideline before its implementation and a similar group of 20 opioid-tolerant patients who were treated according to the new guideline recommendations. Descriptive data included: (1) patient demographics, (2) preoperative opioid and nonopioid use, (3) drug and alcohol history, and (4) preoperative pain scores (**Figs. 5–7**).

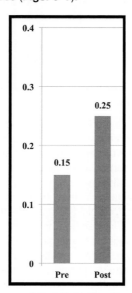

Fig. 5. History of Drug Use in Pre- and Post-Guideline Groups.

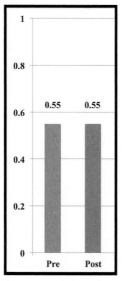

Fig. 6. History of Alcohol Use in Pre- and Post-Guideline Groups.

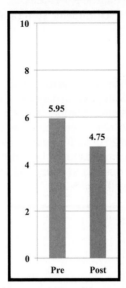

Fig. 7. Preoperative Pain Scores (on a 0 to 10 scale).

Preoperative phase findings included improved identification of opioid-tolerant patients with use of the Pain Screening Tool. Enhanced communication via the EMR and the surgical record resulted in better continuity of care through all phases of the patient's hospitalization. Use of preemptive medications and continuation of chronic pain management medications were also instituted during this phase. The results and improvements are noted in the evaluation of the intraoperative and postoperative phases.

During the intraoperative phase, opioid-tolerant patients were more readily identified. This identification proved critical in alerting caregivers and provided the patient with improved pain management throughout the surgical course. Increased use of multimodal and preemptive analgesics before surgery resulted in improved pain management.

Timely initiation of PCA in the PACU had a positive impact on lowering patient pain scores and led to fewer PCA initiations on the Medical/Surgical Units. Pain ratings in the PACU were improved: mean scores decreased from 3.50 to 0.83 (using a 0 to 10 rating scale). PACU LOS was reduced by approximately 30 minutes (**Figs. 8–10**).

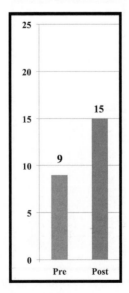

Fig. 8. Use of PCA in PACU.

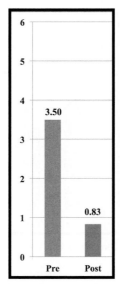

Fig. 9. PACU Pain Scores (on a 0 to 10 scale).

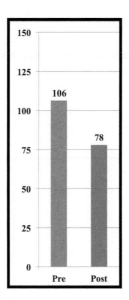

Fig. 10. Minutes in PACU.

Postoperative-phase findings on the Medical/Surgical Units showed improved assessment skills by the nursing staff. Better knowledge about the use of PCA and multimodal pain medications resulted in more timely administration of medication and improved pain management. Continuity of care was improved as PACU handoffs to medical/surgical nurses now included enhanced dialogue about the pain management POC for the opioid-tolerant patient. Improvements included postoperative pain score reduction from a mean of 5.25 to 3.70 (**Fig. 11**).

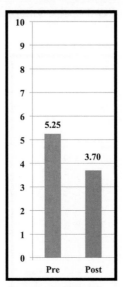

Fig. 11. Postoperative Pain Scores (on a 0 to 10 scale).

Patient education done initially in PEEC was repeated throughout the patient's hospitalization. Preoperative teaching about use of the PCA, assurance of goals for pain control, and mutual agreement about pain scores and management provided better patient understanding and improved their satisfaction with the surgical course. The patient's unrealistic expectation of having no pain postoperatively developed instead into tangible milestones that could be achieved during their hospital stay.

There is good evidence that early physical therapy contributes to earlier discharge.[10] Patients were more cooperative and enthusiastic to work with physical therapy and able to increase their activity because better pain management was achieved. Rehabilitation proceeded faster, as patients with improved pain management were more willing to participate in their activity progression. Hospital LOS decreased by nearly 3 full days (mean of 5.95–3.35) in the guideline population (**Fig. 12**).

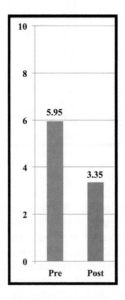

Fig. 12. Hospital LOS (days).

Concern about increasing health care costs prompted the team to quantify the savings that could be realized with guideline implementation. The estimated mean clinical cost savings for the 20 patients in the guideline group was $1650. Extrapolating this dollar figure to the guideline population, it is anticipated that adherence to the new guideline will result in a savings of approximately $100,000 each year (Gary Kienbaum, MSN, Honolulu, HI, personal communication, 2011). Cost savings could be quantified for the patient's stay in the PACU. Improved throughput of patients in the PACU provided a positive impact by reducing wait times for operating room patients seeking PACU admission. Additionally, although not calculated, decreased overtime costs were realized as patient LOS in the PACU was shortened resulting in decreased resource utilization.

Several additional qualitative findings were noted after guideline implementation:

- The Pain Screening Tool showed that it could identify patients who may have been overlooked in the past. Referrals to Pain Service were made at the initial appointment with the surgeon, as opposed to initiating an urgent referral later in the PACU or Medical/Surgical Unit. Although, there was no log of calls before implementation, there were no calls to Pain Service from the PACU after guideline implementation. This avoided a "catch-up" approach when providing patients with pain relief.
- Anecdotal reports from the orthopedic clinic staff showed fewer postoperative clinic and telephone encounters for the group with guideline intervention.
- Before implementation of the guideline, there were transfers to the Skilled Nursing Facility for continued rehabilitation. None of the patients in the guideline group required transfer to the Skilled Nursing Facility for further physical rehabilitation, which may also have impacted cost effectiveness.
- Follow-up phone calls after hospital discharge were recognized as important for assessment and intervention if there were concerns or pain management problems.

LESSONS LEARNED AND RECOMMENDATIONS

Many factors contributed to successful outcomes. These included a team comprising staff in different practice settings, early involvement of key stakeholders including physician participants, an organizational setting that allowed for clinic and inpatient participation in the practice changes, and nursing leadership support for and dedication to promoting the EBP process. Enhanced communication strategies inclusive of a computerized EMR, helped provide seamless information flow for the care of each patient and the project.

Early physician participation was critical to assure that the surgeons and Pain Service physicians would support practice changes. Recognizing key stakeholders and having a clear understanding of their needs helped gain support and proved important to the success of the project. Customization of the Pain Screening Tool made for ease of use and did not prolong the allotted appointment time with the surgeon. Networking and seeking feedback across the continuum of care were beneficial in making process improvements. This networking also raised awareness within the departments of the importance of frequent communication.

Nursing leadership provided encouragement and support that allowed time for development, implementation, and evaluation of the EBP guideline. Strong mentorship was essential to the success of the project. Implementation of an evidence-based project helped encourage professional and personal growth among staff. Enhanced staff education achieved consistency across all practice settings. Early patient education helped patients set realistic expectations about their pain management and increased their satisfaction levels.

Access to librarian support improved team member skills for conducting the literature searches. Identification and utilization of team members with enhanced computer skills proved essential for the project's organization and contributed to minimizing manual workflow processes. Simultaneous access through a shared computer drive provided easy retrieval of the literature reviews, drafts, data, and forms for all team members.

The team was fortunate that no major barriers to progress were encountered. Integral to success was continuous communication between and among team members. Flexibility allowed for adjustments and improvements as the guideline was developed. Some of the challenges included increased utilization of services beyond what was anticipated and untimely format change in the evolving EMR. Improved identification of opioid-tolerant patients led to increased referrals to the Pain Service. This resulted in an increased workload for the Pain Service physicians and emphasized the need to consider the finite nature of current institutional resources.

Cost savings analysis was completed retrospectively. This was an area that could be strengthened through better analysis of the cost savings realized in the various departments. Earlier consultation and preparation with the business analyst would have strengthened the financial analysis of the project.

The successful outcomes achieved by guideline implementation led other surgical services to explore the feasibility of use within their specialties. The Departments of Cardiothoracic and General Surgery have requested to adapt the guideline for their patients. Implementation of an individualized pain management POC showed that it could result in measurably improved patient outcomes.

SUMMARY

The trigger for this EBP project occurred when the Pain Service and Nursing Department noted the difficulties experienced by orthopedic surgical patients with opioid tolerance. The purpose of this project was to identify strategies and develop best practices for pain management in this surgical joint replacement patient population.

Practice changes were implemented across all phases of the surgical experience: preoperative, intraoperative, and postoperative. Patient and clinician participation in developing a pain management POC started at the initial surgical consultation appointment and continued through hospital discharge. Interventions promoted safe and effective pain relief while also optimizing the continuity of care. Use of EBP methodology provided support for intervention development and resulted in meaningful outcomes. This was demonstrated by the ability to enhance quality of care through better patient and staff education, improve patient satisfaction, reduce PACU and hospital LOS, and decrease health care costs.

As increasing numbers of the baby boomer generation seek health care, nursing staff educated in the EBP process can make significant contributions to successful patient outcomes. Health care providers who anticipate the approaching perfect storm in health care and thoughtfully plan, collaborate, and incorporate EBP methods will be well prepared to improve the quality of care, realize cost savings, and meet the challenges ahead.

ACKNOWLEDGMENTS

We would like to acknowledge Dr. Veronica Antoine, Pain Service; Dr. Michael Reyes, Orthopedics; Nursing Administration at Kaiser Moanalua Medical Center and the Hawaii State Center for Nursing for their support and guidance.

REFERENCES

1. Hootman JM, Helmick CG. Projections of US prevalence of arthritis and associated activity limitations. Arthritis Rheum 2006;54(1):226–9.
2. Richebé P, Beaulieu P. Perioperative pain management in the patient treated with. opioids: continuing professional development. Can J Anaesth 2009;56(12): 969–81. http://dx.doi.org/10.1007/s12630-009-9202-y.
3. Kurtz S, Ong K, Lau E, et al. Projections of primary and revision hip and knee arthroplasty in the United States from 2005 to 2030. J Bone Joint Surg Am 2007;89(4):780–5.
4. Carroll IR, Angst MS, Clark JD. Management of perioperative pain in patients chronically consuming opioids. Reg Anesth Pain Med 2004;29(6):576–91.
5. Titler M, Kleiber C, Steelman VJ, et al. The Iowa model of evidence-based practice to promote quality care. Crit Care Nurs Clin North Am 2001;13(4):497–509.
6. Ip HY, Abrishami A, Peng PW, et al. Predictors of postoperative pain and analgesic consumption: a qualitative systematic review. Anesthesiology 2009; 111(3):657–77. http://dx.doi.org/10.1097/ALN.0b013e3181aae87a.
7. American Society of Anesthesiologists Task Force on Acute Pain Management. Practice guidelines for acute pain management in the perioperative setting. Anesthesiology 2012;116(2):248–73. http://dx.doi.org/10.1097/ALN.0b013e18 23c1030.
8. Dalury DF, Lieberman JR, MacDonald SJ. Current and innovative pain management techniques in total knee arthroplasty. J Bone Joint Surg Am 2011;93(20): 1938–43. http://dx.doi.org/10.2106/JBJS.9320icl.
9. Dingley C, Daugherty K, Derieg MK, et al. Improving patient safety through provider communication strategy enhancements. Available at: http://www.ncbi.nlm. nih.gov/books/NBK43663/. Accessed May 26, 2010.
10. Ayalon O, Liu S, Flics S, et al. A multimodal clinical pathway can reduce length of stay after total knee arthroplasty. HSS J 2011;7(1):9–15. http://dx.doi.org/10. 1007/s11420-010-9164-1 Published online 2010 May 22.
11. Carlson CL. Use of three evidence-based postoperative pain assessment practices by registered nurses. Pain Manag Nurs 2009;10(4):174–87. http://dx.doi. org/10.1016/j.pmn.2008.07.001.
12. Gandhi K, Viscusi E. Multimodal pain management techniques in hip and knee arthroplasty. The Journal of the New York School of Regional Anesthesia 2009; 13:1–10.
13. Pasero C, McCaffery M. Orthopaedic postoperative pain management. J Perianesth Nurs 2007;22(3):160–74. http://dx.doi.org/10.1016/j.jopan.2007.02.004.
14. Duellman TJ, Gaffigan C, Milbrandt JC, et al. Multi-modal, Pre-emptive analgesia decreases the length of hospital stay following total joint arthroplasty. Orthopedics 2009;32(3):167. http://dx.doi.org/10.3928/01477447-20090301-08.
15. Dorr LD, Chao L. The emotional state of the patient after total hip and knee arthroplasty. Clin Orthop Relat Res 2007;(463):7–12.
16. Juliano K, Edwards D, Spinello D, et al. Initiating physical therapy on the day of surgery decreases length of stay without compromising functional outcomes following total hip arthroplasty. HSS J 2011;7(1):16–20. http://dx.doi.org/10. 1007/s11420-010-9167-y.

A Simulation Model for Improving Learner and Health Outcomes

Michelle Aebersold, PhD, RN[a],*, Marita G. Titler, PhD, RN, FAAN[b]

KEYWORDS

- Simulation-based learning • Best practices • Learner outcomes • Health outcomes
- Model • Simulation

KEY POINTS

- Simulation-based learning is becoming a necessary component of both prelicensure and postlicensure education and training.
- The research linking simulation-based learning and patient outcomes is largely underdeveloped.
- Simulation-based learning needs to be grounded in the science of learning.

Simulation-based learning is a necessary component of teaching in the health sciences, both in prelicensure training and postlicensure competency development, ongoing education, training, and evaluation. Simulation is an integral component in both military and aviation training. Nursing and medicine use sophisticated computerized mannequins and virtual environments that support learning in the health sciences; schools and universities are investing significant dollars in both infrastructure and technology to support the growing trend in simulation-based learning. It is becoming imperative that simulation-based learning is grounded in the theoretic foundations and science of learning and, although much work has already been done in this area, more work is needed.

To support continued research on the impact of simulation-based education and learning, the authors have developed a model of simulation-based learning, the Simulation Model for Improving Learner and Health Outcomes (SMILHO) described herein. The framework set forth focuses on concepts that embody the best evidence on how learners (students and clinicians) effectively develop new knowledge and skills to use in their practice. One goal of this framework is to improve health outcomes, both

Disclosures: None.

[a] Division of Systems Leadership and Effectiveness Science, University of Michigan School of Nursing, Room 4156, 400 North Ingalls Building, Ann Arbor, MI 48109-5482, USA; [b] Division of Systems Leadership and Effectiveness Science, University of Michigan School of Nursing, Room 4170, 400 North Ingalls Building, Ann Arbor, MI 48109-5482, USA

* Corresponding author.

E-mail address: mabersol@med.umich.edu

patient and population health, by ensuring clinicians practice at a high level of competence that is based on the best available evidence for specified phenomena (eg, prevention of falls, interdisciplinary communication, and handoffs). This framework was developed based on current learning theories, known research in simulation-based learning, and upon the authors' research and application of these theories. The framework is intended to guide the use of simulation-based learning to improve learner outcomes and health outcomes. SMILHO can be applied to many different types of simulation-based learning in the educational and practice setting, as well as measure the impact on learner and health outcomes. The purpose of this article is to introduce the SMILHO framework, describe its components, and present an exemplar to demonstrate how the reader might use the framework in simulation-based learning.

BACKGROUND

Simulation is defined as the artificial replication of a real-world environment in which learners interact with objects/technology to learn evidence-based processes of care and achieve specific learning outcomes.[1] Simulation techniques can be designed in a variety of ways and use a variety of technologies matched to achieve the best learning experience. For example, the experience could involve using a high-fidelity (computer-driven) mannequin simulator in which the learning outcomes involve an increase in decision making to provide evidence-based care to sepsis patients using evidence-based care bundles. As learners use evidence-based practices (EBPs) during simulation, the outcomes of the simulated patient improve.[2] The experience could also be a role-play simulation technique in a virtual world in which the learner (represented as an avatar) practices his or her communication and delegation skills to develop more effective skills in managing a clinical situation.[3] Another example might use computerized unfolding case studies in which the learner is exposed to the impact of his or her decisions on a patient's risk of developing a urinary tract infection. Those decisions would include determining the appropriate time to discontinue a Foley catheter and begin a toileting program.

Simulation is well integrated into many health science education programs, including medicine and nursing.[1,4–6] It is also used in many practice-related areas such as triage, cardiac arrests, patient deterioration, and collaborative team training.[7–13] Early simulation studies focused primarily on learner outcomes measured during or immediately after the simulation-based learning experience. They generally measured knowledge and skill acquisition and learner satisfaction with the experience or self-perception of his or her improved confidence or self-efficacy levels. Although these variables are important to measure, they fall short of evaluating the real impact that simulation can have: transfer of skills and knowledge from the learning environment to the patient care environment and the impact on patient outcomes.

Evaluation of the impact of simulation-based learning on patient care outcomes creates several challenges. Often the impact of the skills and knowledge acquired during the simulation are not easily measured in the patient care environment. It is difficult to measure improvement in critical thinking skills without extensive direct observation of learners in practice settings. New studies are emerging that are measuring patient outcomes; however this early research has primarily targeted the impact of team training, mock codes, and specific task training such as surgical skills on patient safety and/or patient outcomes.[7,11,12,14–16] Many of these studies have evaluated physicians or teams of physicians and nurses, and few studies have focused on the direct impact of nursing on patient outcomes. Thus, research regarding the impact of simulation on patient and health outcomes is still largely underdeveloped.

MODEL DEVELOPMENT

SMILHO (**Fig. 1**) focuses on the science of learning applied in simulation to align clinician and student practice behaviors with research evidence to improve health outcomes of patients and populations. The model set forth herein focuses on concepts that embody the best evidence on how learners (students and clinicians) effectively transfer learned knowledge and skills into their practice. One goal of this model is to improve health outcomes by ensuring clinicians practice at a high level of competence that is based on the best available evidence for specified phenomena (eg, prevention of falls, interdisciplinary communication, and handoffs). This model was developed based on current theories of effective learning, the authors' research in simulation-based learning, and research by other investigators in this field of science.[2,3,17–24]

The simulation component of the model embodies 3 central concepts critical to the use of simulation as a learning technique: learning event, active engagement, and debriefing. Together, these concepts guide the design and delivery of simulation-based learning to improve practice behaviors with the ultimate goal of improving health care outcomes. The outcomes component of the model focuses on 2 areas, learner outcomes and health outcomes at the patient and population level. Each of these concepts (learning event, active engagement, debriefing, learner outcomes, and health outcomes) are described in the following sections.

LEARNING EVENT

The first concept in the SMILHO model is the development of the learning experience in which the learner engages. This concept is called the learning event. It is grounded in part on the work by Kolb,[21] Ericsson,[19,20] and Aldrich,[24] and expanded, based on

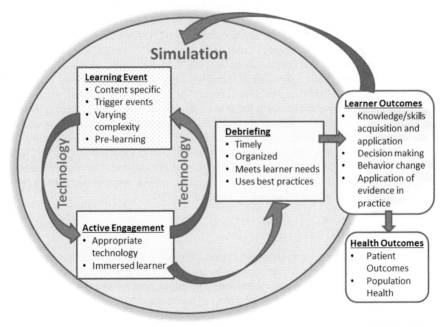

© Michelle Aebersold

Fig. 1. A simulation model to improve learner and health outcomes (SMILHO). (*Courtesy of* M. Aebersold, Ann Arbor, MI.)

the authors' work, to develop the entire experience. The determination of the learning event establishes the basis for the instructional andragogy and the selection of the learning technologies utilized. Therefore the learning event becomes the experience that the learner engages in and is embedded within an overall simulation experience. This learning event allows the learner to engage in experiential learning, which has an impact on the effectiveness of the learning. It is content specific, meaning that it is designed with clear objectives around a specific content area (eg, fall prevention or communication). This content is aligned with the specific outcome (eg, behavior change, knowledge and/or skill acquisition and application, decision making skill, or application of evidence) that is desired. The focus is generally on improving procedural knowledge, knowing how and when to apply knowledge learned.[25]

The learning event varies in complexity depending on the learner needs and the goals and objectives. Higher-level skills will likely need a more complex learning event than lower-level skills. The number of skills to be learned will also drive the complexity. Learners who are applying a set of patient-specific evidence-based practices may need a series of simulations or case studies to meet the learning objectives, whereas first-level nursing students needing to learn a basic skill may only need a simple case scenario with a low-level task trainer such as a catheterization simulator.

The learning event also needs trigger events to elicit the particular behaviors or decisions the learner needs to practice. They can include changes in patient vital signs, new information presented in the scenario, or decision points. Trigger events can be designed using a framework such as The Event Based Approach to Training,[26] or methods such as branching storylines used in game designs.[24] A novice learner may need more obvious triggers to elicit the desired behavior during early experiences.

There are several models that can be used to design the learning event. Aebersold and Tschannen[27] developed a 5-step approach to simulation development that can be used to guide the development of both virtual and mannequin-based simulation, and ensures alignment with core competencies such as Quality and Safety Education for Nurses (QSEN).[28] Jeffries[29] addresses simulation design characteristics in her simulation framework, including fidelity, cues, and complexity, which can be used for designing simulations and evaluations. Aldrich,[24] in his book on simulations and serious games, has many examples of immersive games and simulations.

The learning event also requires some amount of pre-learning or preparation on the learner's part to ensure the learning experience is effective. This pre-learning will help the learner be prepared to participate more fully in the actual learning event and can include the use of podcasts, reading materials, or virtual communities. It may also include a review of the procedures he or she will use during the simulation. Then the learner applies that knowledge in a true-to-life clinical experience. The amount of pre-learning is determined based on the level of the learner, the complexity of the learning experience, and the desired outcomes.

ACTIVE ENGAGEMENT

The active engagement component promotes effective active learning. In this component, the appropriate type of technology is specified and is selected specifically to meet the objectives and goals in the learning event and to ensure the learner is immersed, meaning that his or her attention is completely focused on and within the experience. An example is when a high-fidelity simulator allows the learner to be completely immersed in a patient simulation to achieve the objectives of learning how to direct a code team, whereas learning how to place an intravenous (IV) catheter might be best accomplished using a virtual IV trainer. Gaba,[1] in his article on the future vision of simulation, stresses the importance of selecting the right technology to meet the goal of the simulation. This will become increasingly important as simulation begins to play a central role in the education of health care practitioners. It will be important to not only select the right technology to promote learner immersion, but also to evaluate the effectiveness of the technology used in the simulation both from for validity and reliability of the simulator[30] as well as to compare technology-enhanced simulation with other instructional methods.[31]

DEBRIEFING

Debriefing has become an essential component of simulation-based learning. It is the process in which the learner reviews the experience and develops an understanding of what occurred and what was learned from the experience. It is often based on the principles of reflective practice[22,32] and is a critical component and the place where much of the learning occurs, and changes are integrated into future behaviors. This facilitated conversation is timely and occurs after an event, either real or simulated, in which the participants review what occurred and analyze their actions, emotions, and thought processes.

The debriefing process should be highly organized and needs to occur in a manner to allow for a safe environment in which learners are allowed to reflect and grow from the experience and should be designed to meet the needs of the learners. The facilitator of the debriefing sessions needs to be trained in appropriate facilitation methods and should use best practices in debriefing. The International Nursing Association of Clinical Simulation and Learning (INACSL) has published Standards of Best Practices in Simulation, including those on debriefing.[33] If managed poorly, the debriefing experience can leave learners with misinformation and feelings of low self-efficacy or erroneous learning and uncorrected poor critical thinking.[34] Debriefing helps learners to make connections between the simulated experience and other clinical experiences they have encountered.[21,22] This assists learners to create a context or perspective based on their experiences and supports the theory of experiential learning.[21]

Various methods are available to guide debriefing in a structured and effective manner.[35–38] Consistently, the methods recommended include:

1. Learners' reflection of their actions
2. Engaging discussions
3. Learners' reflection on mental models used in their decision making
4. Examination of clinical reasoning guided by nursing diagnosis and care priorities
5. Exploration of performance gaps and ways in which the learners' mental models may contribute to these gaps
6. Short lectures in which experts share suggestions on how learners might approach the situation in the future to obtain a better outcomes

LEARNER OUTCOMES

Outcomes in this model focus on learner outcomes and health outcomes. Learner outcomes are the specific learner proficiencies or changes in behavior that are achieved as a result of the simulation-based learning experience (learning event, active engagement, and debriefing). Learner outcomes measured are generally an increase in knowledge or skill acquisition and application, improved decision making, behavior change, and application of evidence in practice. Learner outcomes are both the drivers of the learning and behavior change and results of the learning experience. Desired outcomes must be specified first to support the design of the learning experience and influence the learning event, active engagement, and debriefing. Then the desired learner outcomes must be evaluated to determine if the learning experience was effective. This can be a challenging part of the simulation-based learning process but is critically important as research in simulation-based learning moves forward. Most commonly, this evaluation is done as part of the simulation-based learning event. Learners can be given knowledge tests after engaging in the experience to measure knowledge acquisition, or their skills can be evaluated in subsequent simulations or in actual clinical performance to determine skill application. It is more difficult to measure the application of decision-making skills, but this can be done by engaging learners in a simulation-based experience designed to measure those skills or in after-action reports of events such as a cardiac arrest in which performance is generally reviewed. The use of EBP can be measured during simulation[2] or evaluated in the clinical environment through observation or chart reviews. Kirkpartick's[39] 4 levels of evaluating training programs are useful and can be applied to simulation-based learning; Schaefer and colleagues[30] found a large number of studies looking at translation of impact of simulation into the patient care environment used Kirkpatrick's levels.

The feedback loop from outcomes back to simulation-based learning depicts learners' building their knowledge and experiences from 1 simulation to the next over time. This becomes the basis for more complex or novel simulations in which the learner can continue to learn by applying what he or she knows to future simulations. Experiential learning is described by Kolb[21] as a learning cycle. In this cycle, learners have a concrete experience, reflect upon that experience, develop an abstract conceptualization of the experience, and then move to test that through active experimentation. To become experts in a given field or practice area, learners must engage in experiential learning to develop solid practice behaviors that support safe and effective patient care. This also supports Ericsson's[19,20] theory of deliberate practice, in which learners engage in goal-directed repeated practice of skills. In this way, the learners continue to build their expertise and ability to problem solve situations to support safe and effective patient care. This also supports continuous or lifelong learning patterns in individuals.

HEALTH OUTCOMES

Health outcomes include both patient outcomes and population outcomes; they comprise a critically important part of this model yet are the most difficult to measure. It is essential, however, that one understands how simulation-based learning can impact the health outcomes of patients and populations served by health care providers. Capturing the impact of simulation on health outcomes is a major challenge for future researchers in simulation-based learning. Learner behaviors and skills can be measured, but do they impact the health outcomes of patients? In certain areas referenced earlier, patient outcomes have been measured with good success; however, as stated, the ability to measure patient outcomes in many areas is undeveloped. Zigmont and colleagues[40] state for simulation education to be sustainable, a link to patient outcomes is needed. This can be done by first identifying the specific health outcomes that are being targeted by the simulation experience and then developing metrics to evaluate those. For example, if one is trying to improve nurse to health care provider communication to reduce communication errors and improve patient safety, then one could measure the number of adverse patient incidents that occur as a result of communication errors.

EXEMPLAR

To achieve the objective of improving the use of structured communication tools (content) and increasing the effectiveness of nurse to health care provider communication, the learner (in this case a student nurse) would first learn about a specific structured communication tool used in nursing crew resource management (NCRM), the 3W's.[41] This pre-learning might occur as a self-learning module or didactic presentation and could include some initial role play. Then the learner would engage in the simulation designed to recreate a situation in which the learner must effectively use the structured communication tool (3W's) to deliver optimal care to the patient and therefore produce a positive patient outcome. The simulation objectives support the use of the structured communication tool, and the triggers (the patient experiences a sudden decline) prompt the learner to engage in a discussion with a health care provider to obtain appropriate orders and treatments for the patient. Only when the structured communication tool (3W's) is used effectively will the learner receive the needed treatment orders from the health care provider and see improvement in the simulated patient. The active engagement occurs through the appropriate use of a high-fidelity mannequin (eg, Sim Man 3G-Laerdal [Laerdal Medical, Wappingers Falls, NY, USA]) to ensure the learner stays immersed with the scenario and is able to monitor the patient's responses to treatments. Debriefing occurs immediately after the scenario and is organized around a discussion of the communication that occurred between the student and the health care provider; it includes a discussion of the 3W's (meeting the learner's needs). It uses a reflective debriefing approach and is facilitated by a trained facilitator (best practice). The learner outcomes are measured using a tool to capture how well the student is able to recognize the patient condition (situational awareness), uses the 3W's, and makes decisions about how to respond.[17] This exemplar only goes through learner outcomes. It is challenging to link student outcomes to health outcomes; however, if this was done with nurses, one could measure adverse outcomes in patients linked to nurse/provider communication incidents.

SUMMARY

Simulation has become a necessary and integral part of education for both prelicensure and ongoing education of health care practitioners. To guide this process, the SMILHO model provides a framework to design the experience from a science of learning approach and links it to both learner and health outcomes to add to the knowledge base on simulation-based learning's impact on outcomes. Much work has been done in this area, and the SMILHO model will support the future work needed to continue to create effective simulation-based learning experiences and move simulation-based research from knowledge and skill evaluation to learner and health outcomes.

REFERENCES

1. Gaba DM. The future vision of simulation in health care. Qual Saf Health Care 2004;13(Suppl 1):i2–10.
2. Aebersold M. Using simulation to improve the use of evidence-based practice guidelines. West J Nurs Res 2011;33(3):296–305.
3. Tschannen D, Aebersold M, McLaughlin E, et al. Use of virtual simulations for improving knowledge transfer among baccalaureate nursing students. J Nurs Educ Pract 2012;2(3):15–24.

4. Cannon-Diehl MR. Simulation in healthcare and nursing: state of the science. Crit Care Nurs Q 2009;32(2):128–36.

5. Issenberg SB, McGaghie WC, Petrusa ER, et al. Features and uses of high-fidelity medical simulations that lead to effective learning: a BEME systematic review. Med Teach 2005;27(1):10–28.

6. Nehring WM, Lashley FR. Nursing simulation: a review of the past 40 years. Simul Gaming 2009;40:528–52.

7. Andreatta P, Saxton E, Thompson M, et al. Simulation-based mock codes significantly correlate with improved pediatric patient cardiopulmonary arrest survival rates. Pediatr Crit Care Med 2011;12(1):33–8.

8. Endacott R, Scholes J, Cooper S, et al. Identifying patient deterioration: using simulation and reflective interviewing to examine decision making skills in a rural hospital. Int J Nurs Stud 2012;49(6):710–7.

9. Kardon-Edgren S, Adamson KA. BSN medical–surgical student ability to perform CPR in a simulation: recommendations and implications. Clinical Simulation in Nursing 2009;5(2):e79–83.

10. Messmer PR. Enhancing nurse–physician collaboration using pediatric simulation. J Contin Educ Nurs 2008;39(7):319–27.

11. Phipps MG, Lindquist DG, McConaughey E, et al. Outcomes from a labor and delivery team training program with simulation component. Am J Obstet Gynecol 2011;206(1):3–9.

12. Riley W, Davis S, Miller K, et al. Didactic and simulation nontechnical skills team training to improve perinatal patient outcomes in a community hospital. Jt Comm J Qual Patient Saf 2011;37(8):357–64.

13. Wolf L. The use of human patient simulation in ED triage training can improve nursing confidence and patient outcomes. J Emerg Nurs 2008;34(2):169–71.

14. Wayne DB, Didwania A, Feinglass J, et al. Simulation-based education improves quality of care during cardiac arrest team responses at an academic teaching hospital: a case–control study. Chest 2008;133(1):56–61.

15. Zendejas B, Brydges R, Wang AT, et al. Patient outcomes in simulation-based medical education: a systematic review. J Gen Intern Med 2013;28(8):1078–89.

16. Shea-Lewis A. Teamwork: crew resource management in a community hospital. J Healthc Qual 2009;31(5):14–8.

17. Aebersold M, Tschannen D, Sculli G. Improving nursing students' communication skills using crew resource management strategies. J Nurs Educ 2013;52(3):125–30.

18. Aebersold M. Capacity to rescue: nurse behaviors that rescue patients [Unpublished Dissertation]. University of Michigan; 2008. Available at: http://hdl.handle.net/2027.42/60718.

19. Ericsson KA. Deliberate practice and the acquisition and maintenance of expert performance in medicine and related domains. Acad Med 2004;79(Suppl 10):S70–81.

20. Ericsson KA. Deliberate practice and acquisition of expert performance: a general overview. Acad Emerg Med 2008;15(11):988–94.

21. Kolb DA. Experiential learning: experience as the source of learning and development. Upper Saddle River (NJ): Prentice-Hall, Inc; 1984.

22. Schon DA. The reflective practitioner: how professionals think in action. San Francisco (CA): Jossey Bass; 1983.

23. Tschannen D, Aebersold M, Sauter C, et al. Improving nurses' perceptions of competency in diabetes self-management education through the use of simulation and problem-based learning. J Contin Educ Nurs 2013;44(6):257–63.

24. Aldrich C. The complete guide to simulation and serious games. San Francisco (CA): John Wiley & Sons; 2009.

25. Krathwahl DR. A revision of Bloom's taxonomy: an overview. Theory Pract 2002; 41(4):213–64.
26. Rosen MA, Salas E, Wu TS, et al. Promoting teamwork: an event-based approach to simulation-based teamwork training for emergency medicine residents. Acad Emerg Med 2008;15(11):1190–8.
27. Aebersold M, Tschannen D. Virtual reality simulations: teaching interpersonal and clinical judgment skills to healthcare practitioners. In: Cruz-Cunha MM, editor. Handbook of research on serious games as education, business, research tools. Hershey (PA): IGI Global; 2012. p. 800–17.
28. Cronenwett L, Sherwood G, Barnsteiner J, et al. Quality and safety education for nurses. Nurs Outlook 2007;55(3):122–31.
29. Jeffries PR. A framework for designing, implementing, and evaluating simulations used as teaching strategies in nursing. Nurs Educ Perspect 2005;26(2):96–103.
30. Schaefer JJ, Vanderbilt AA, Cason CL, et al. Literature review: instructional design and pedagogy science in healthcare simulation. Simul Healthc 2011;6(Suppl): S30–41.
31. Cook DA, Brydges R, Zendejas B, et al. Technology-enhanced simulation to assess health professionals: a systematic review of validity evidence, research methods and reporting quality. Acad Med 2013;88(6):1–10.
32. Rudolph JW, Simon R, Dufresne RL, et al. There's no such thing as "nonjudgmental" debriefing: a theory and method for debriefing with good judgment. Simulation in Healthcare 2006;1(1):49–55.
33. Decker S, Fey M, Sideras S, et al. Standards of best practice: simulation standard IV: the debriefing process. Clinical Simulation in Nursing 2013;9:e26–9.
34. Dreifuerst KT. The essentials of debriefing in simulation learning: a concept analysis. Nurs Educ Perspect 2009;30(2):109–14.
35. Brett-Fleegler M, Rudolph J, Eppich W, et al. Debriefing assessment for simulation in healthcare: development and psychometric properties. Simul Healthc 2012;7(5):288–94.
36. Kuiper R, Heinrich C, Matthias A, et al. Debriefing with the OPT model of clinical reasoning during high fidelity patient simulation. Int J Nurs Educ Scholarsh 2008; 5:17. http://dx.doi.org/10.2202/1548-923X.1466.
37. Rudolph JW, Simon R, Raemer DB, et al. Debriefing as formative assessment: closing performance gaps in medical education. Acad Emerg Med 2008; 15(11):1010–6.
38. Rudolph JW, Simon R, Rivard P, et al. Debriefing with good judgment: combining rigorous feedback with genuine inquiry. Anesthesiol Clin 2007;25(2):361–76.
39. Kirkpatrick DL. Evaluating training programs: the four levels. San Francisco (CA): Berrett-Koehler; 1994.
40. Zigmont JJ, Kappus L, Sudikoff SN. The 3D model of debriefing: defusing, discovering, and deepening. Semin Perinatol 2011;35(2):52–8.
41. Sculli GL, Sine DM. Soaring to success: taking crew resource management from the cockpit to the nursing unit. Danvers (MA): HCPro; 2011.

Index

Note: Page numbers of article titles are in **boldface** type.

A

Acute cervical spinal cord injury. *See* Cervical spinal cord injury.
Agitated patients, reducing restraint use in trauma center emergency room, **371–381**

B

Behavioral health, reducing restraint use in trauma center emergency room, **371–381**
Brain injury, normothermia for neuroprotection in patients with, **399–413**
    evaluation, 407–408
        monitoring practice change, 407–408
        nursing compliance, 408
    evidence for practice improvement, 400–402
        assemble, critique, and synthesize literature, 401–402
        forming a team, 401
        knowledge and problem triggers, 400–401
    implementation strategies, 402–407
        development of guideline, 401–404
        educational strategies and marketing, 405–407
        impact of shivering, 404
    lessons learned, 408–410

C

Cervical spinal cord injury, acute, pulmonary management of patients with, **357–369**
    evaluation, 365–366
    evidence for practice improvement, 359–363
    implementation strategies, 363–365
    lessons learned, 366–367
Cognitive impairment, pain identification in nursing home residents with, **345–356**
    evaluation, 352–353
    evidence for practice improvement, 346–350
    implementation strategies, 350–352
    lessons learned, 353–355

D

Delirium, promoting sleep in adult surgical intensive care unit to prevent, **383–397**
    evaluation, 391–395
    evidence for practice improvement, 386–387
    formation of a team, 385–386
    implementation strategies, 387–391
    lessons learned, 395–396

Nurs Clin N Am 49 (2014) 441–452
http://dx.doi.org/10.1016/S0029-6465(14)00054-1
0029-6465/14/$ – see front matter © 2014 Elsevier Inc. All rights reserved.

nursing.theclinics.com